SIRTFOOD DIET COOKBOOK

302 Quick and Healthy Sirtfood Diet Recipes to Use in Your Meal Plan.

Discover the Power of Sirtuins: Activate the Metabolism, Eat Delicious

Dishes and Lose Weight Quickly

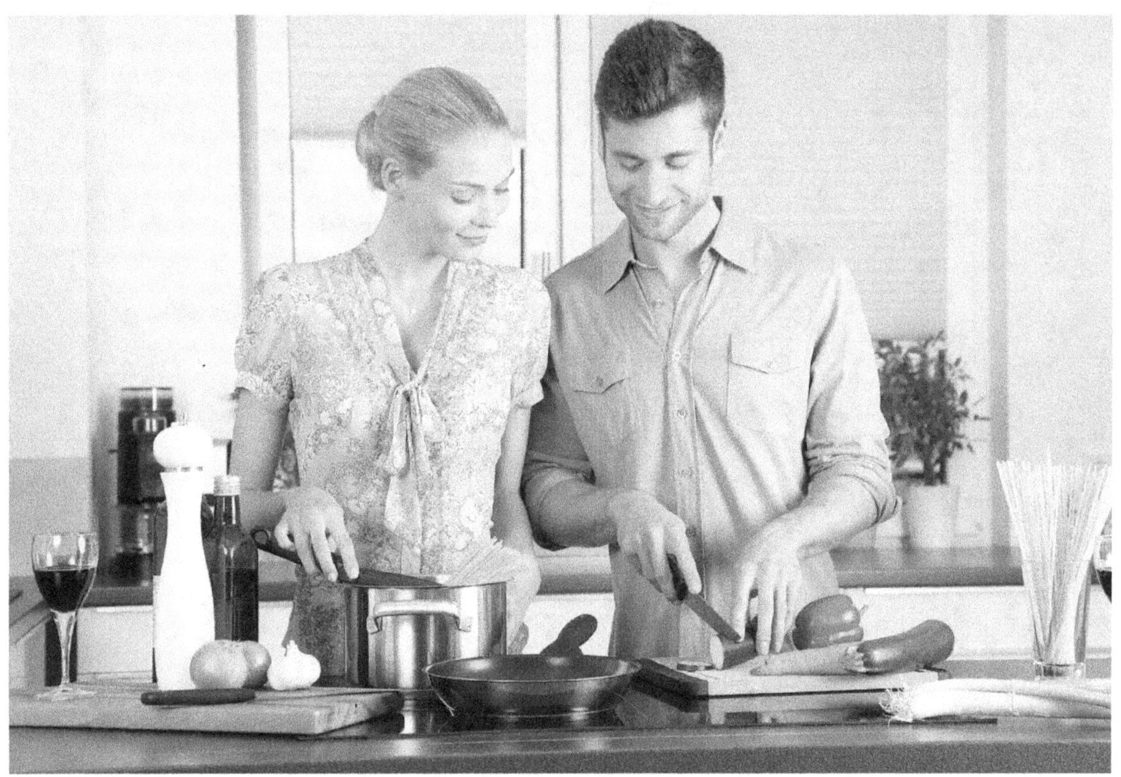

Lara Burns

Table of Contents

Introduction

Sirtfood diet is a new effective method for weight loss and helps the body regenerate. Sirtfood diet is a combination of fresh, low-fat foods that contain sirtuins and tiny organisms such as microalgae, yeast, and bacteria. According to the study prepared by the American Society for nutrition, sirtuins improve the health of people and can help slow the aging process. The diet includes foods that contain a natural antioxidant called nicotinamide riboside (NR). Sirtuin food is found in a wide range of specific products like berries, avocado, blackcurrants, grapes, parsley, grapefruit, lemon peel and kale. Sirtuins can turn genes on or off and raise the level of enzymes that destroy damaged proteins. The study also suggests that these types of food can help in a weight-loss program and can protect body cells from stress.

About 'Sirtfood Diet'

Sirtfood diet is the latest breakthrough, natural diet. The natural diet is enriched with all the nutrients that aid weight loss and reduce the risk of serious diseases. The Sirtfood diet incorporates various foods that are rich in antioxidants, polyphenols and fatty acids. The natural diet helps to achieve weight loss, cure chronic and general illness and improve overall health. Hence this method is called the 'Sirtfood diet.' There are many health benefits of the Sirtfood diet, which are told by dietitians in this blog. The sirtfood diet has been proved that it enhances longevity and also promote sleep for rejuvenating the body because of other nutrients included in the food. The diet incorporates exceptional foods ideally a diverse selection of polyphenols and other molecules that act to improve your nutrition with a special ingredient called Sirtuin Activators (STA's). The diet also combats diseases like Alzheimer's and other chronic ailments.

What is Sirtfood Diet?

'Sirtfood diet' is a new weight-loss diet plan consisting of foods that are rich in natural antioxidants and polyphenols. These foods enhance the production of a chemical known as 'Sirtuin'. Sirtuin helps in the formation of proteins and helps slow down the process of aging. The antioxidant and polyphenol-rich food is also believed to reduce the risks of cancer and other critical diseases. So, the sirtfood diet is an ideal diet for reducing weight and preventing disease. These foods usually boost sirtuin levels, which in turn produce the protein resveratrol, that is known to reduce the risk of age-related diseases. Moreover, resveratrol can also stop the processes of aging. This is what we call diet with maximum sirtuin activators. The diet has the power to boost weight loss, it also has multiple health benefits.

How does the Sirtfood diet works?

The sirtfood diet works by aiming to boost levels of a chemical called Sirtuin. Research has found that eating foods that boost Sirtuin levels aids weight loss, can also help fight diseases like cancer, help improve sleep and cure metabolic disorders. This chemical is activated by a molecule called Sirtuin Activators (STA's) present in various foods. The Sirtfood diet consists of foods rich in Sirtuin Activators (STA's) like Sirtfoods. These foods include berries, avocado, blackcurrants, grapes, parsley, grapefruit, lemon peel, kale, etc. The Sirtfood diet consists of anti-inflammatory, anti-oxidant rich foods that also include minimum calories to reduce weight. Sirt supplements can also be taken externally to improve results. Overall, the sirtfood diet helps calorie restriction, reduce weight, and also maintain overall health.

Sirtfoods - the best part of the Sirtfood diet

The sirtfoods are the main part of the diet. Most of the foods are rich in a powerful antioxidant called 'Sirtuin.' Sirtuin has the ability to change cellular metabolic processes and regulations. The mitochondrion is a part of our cells. Normally mitochondria are active and help in energy production. As we grow older, these mitochondria become damaged and are not able to function properly. The sirtuin works by scavenging the free radicals and stabilizing the mitochondrial to work properly again. This helps to increase cellular metabolism by improving energy production. With this increased production of energy, people are able to boost their metabolism, thereby giving good health and good health. In addition to this, Sirtuin also acts as a protective shield by stopping the attack of free radicals by DNA, proteins, and lipids, and this protects them from oxidative damage. However, there are no definite statistics on the role of Sirtuin on human health. The studies are ongoing to determine the precise mechanism of the functions of Sirtuin on human health. However, the health benefits of Sirtuin have been observed.

Benefits of Sirtfood diet

Yes, the Sirtfood diet is actually a leading weight loss diet, which aims for rapid weight loss in a short span of time. Research has indicated that it will also help in reducing appetite, prevent diseases, improve sleep, and also boost energy.

Weight loss - Based on long-term research, it appears that eating Sirtfoods can help reduce your weight. According to research by a team of scientists from the University of Eastern Finland, people who were on a diet lost an average of 12 pounds in 14 weeks. Laboratory mice eating sirtfoods showed an increase in calorie-burning cell function. Women taking the sirtfood diet had increased fat burning ability while those in the control group did not.

Cardiovascular Disease - Scientists have suggested that the intake of sirtfoods may help lower the risk of heart attacks, stroke and other cardiovascular diseases.

Brain Health - Sirtfoods have been found to increase the levels of acetylcholine, which plays an important role in Alzheimer's and dementia.

Metabolic Syndrome - This condition is common among many people though it does not result in any major health issues. However, some studies have established that eating sirtfoods may lead to a reduction in 'Metabolic Syndrome'.

Diabetes - A study conducted by the University of Eastern Finland has indicated that people on the sirtfoods lost two-thirds of body weight within two weeks. The researchers noted that those people who lost the most weight were those who followed the diet for two weeks longer than the other group of individuals in the study.

Anti-aging - Sirtfoods have been found to have anti-aging properties. Research has indicated that eating sirtfoods helps lower the risk of age-related diseases like osteoporosis and colon cancer. In addition, it is being considered that since sirtfoods is an antioxidant, eating them can also help fight off certain cancers, such as those of the prostate or breast.

Oxidation - The Sirtfood diet can help decrease cellular oxidation caused by free radicals. It can also reduce the molecular damage which is caused by free radicals by repairing the damage to DNA and proteins. It was found in a study conducted by researchers in Milan, Italy, that the diet can reduce the oxidized by 60% while a control diet has no effect on it.

Aging - The Sirtfood diet helps prevent cellular aging. In addition, it pays backward and encourages the production of new youthful energy throughout the entire body.

Sirtfood Diet

The basis of the sirtuin diet can be explained in simple terms or complex ways. However, it is crucial to understand how and why it works to appreciate what you are doing. It is essential also to know why these sirtuin rich foods help you maintain fidelity to your diet plan. Otherwise, you may throw something in your meal with less nutrition that would defeat the purpose of planning for one rich in sirtuins. Most importantly, this is not a dietary fad, and as you will see, there is much wisdom in how humans have used natural foods, even for medicinal purposes, over thousands of years.

To understand how the Sirtfood diet works and why these particular foods are necessary, we will look at their role in the human body.

Sirtuin activity was first researched in yeast, where a mutation caused an extension in the yeast's lifespan. Sirtuins were also shown to slow aging in laboratory mice, fruit flies, and nematodes. As Sirtuins' research proved to transfer to mammals, they were examined for their diet and slowing the aging process. The sirtuins in humans are different in typing, but they essentially work in the same ways and reasons.

There are seven "members" that establish the sirtuin family. It is believed that sirtuins play a significant role in regulating certain functions of cells, including proliferation (reproduction and growth of cells), apoptosis (death of cells). They promote survival and resist stress to increase longevity.

They are also seen to block neurodegeneration (loss of function of the brain's nerve cells). They conduct their housekeeping functions by cleaning out toxic proteins and supporting the brain's ability to change and adapt to different conditions or recuperate (i.e., brain plasticity). As part of this, they also help reduce chronic inflammation and reduce so-called oxidative stress. It happens when there are too many cell-damaging free radicals circulating in the body, and the body cannot catch up by combating them with antioxidants. These factors are related to age-related illness and weight, which again brings us back to discussing how they work.

You will see labels in Sirtuins that start with "SIR," representing "Silence Information Regulator" genes. They do precisely that, silence or regulate, as part of their functions. The seven sirtuins humans work with are SIRT1, SIRT2, SIRT3, SIRT4, SIRT 5, SIRT6and SIRT7. Each of these types is responsible for different areas of protecting cells. They work by either stimulating or turning on certain gene expressions or reducing and turning off other gene expressions. This essentially means that they can influence genes to do more or less of something, most of which they are already programmed to do.

Through enzyme reactions, each of the SIRT types affects different cells responsible for the metabolic processes that help maintain life. This is also related to what organs and functions they will affect.

For example, the SIRT6 causes and expression of genes in humans affect skeletal muscle, fat tissue, brain, and heart. SIRT 3 would cause an expression of genes that affect the kidneys, liver, brain, and heart.

If we tie these concepts together, you can see that the Sirtuin proteins can change the expression of genes and in the case of the Sirtfood Diet, we care about how sirtuins can turn off those genes that are responsible for speeding up aging and for weight management.

The other aspect to this conversation of sirtuins is the function and the power of calorie restriction on the human body. Calorie restriction is only eating fewer calories. This, coupled with exercise and reducing stress, is usually a combination of weight loss. Calorie restriction has also proven across much research in animals and humans to increase one's lifespan.

We can look further at the role of sirtuins with calorie restriction and using the SIRT3 protein, which has a role in metabolism and aging. Amongst all of the effects of the protein on gene expression (such as preventing cells from dying, reducing tumors from growing, etc.), we want to understand the effects of SIRT3 on weight for this manuscript.

As we stated earlier, the SIRT3 has high expression in those metabolically active tissues, and its ability to express itself increases with caloric restriction, fasting, and exercise. On the contrary, it will express itself less when the body has high fat, high-calorie-riddled diet.

The last few highlights of sirtuins are their role in regulating telomeres and reducing inflammation, which also helps prevent disease and aging.

Telomeres are sequences of proteins at the ends of chromosomes. When cells divide, these get shorter. As we age, they get shorter and other stressors to the body also will contribute to this.

Maintaining these longer telomeres is the key to slower aging. Also, proper diet, along with exercise and other variables, can lengthen telomeres. SIRT6 is one of the sirtuins that, if activated, can help with DNA damage, inflammation and oxidative stress. SIRT1 also helps with inflammatory response cycles that are related to many age-related diseases.

Calories restriction, as we mentioned earlier, can extend life to some degree.

Since this and fasting are a stressor, these factors will stimulate the SIRT3 proteins to kick in and protect the body from the stressors and excess free radicals. Again, the telomere length is affected as well.

To sum up, all of this information also shows that, contrary to some people's beliefs, genetics, like "it is what it is" or "it is my fate because Uncle Joe has something…" through our own lifestyle choices. What we are exposed to, we can influence action and changes in our genes. This is quite an empowering thought and yet another reason why you should be excited to have a science-based diet such as the Sirtfood diet, available to you.

Having laid this all out before you, you should be able to appreciate how and why these miraculous compounds work in your favor to keep you youthful, healthy and lean. If they are working hard for you, don't you feel that you should do something too?

Lara Burns

Benefits of Sirtfood Diet

The Sirtuins

Sirtuins are a group of seven proteins that maintain cell metabolism and homeostasis at optimal levels. Three of these proteins are found in the mitochondria, one is in the cytoplasm, and another three are located in the nucleus. Sirtuins maintain the cell's health and ensure that all processes going on within the cell are correctly happening. Sirtuins can, however, not be effective without the presence of NAD+ (nicotinamide adenine dinucleotide). NAD+ is a coenzyme that is present in all cells that are living in nature. NAD+ ensures that Sirtuins function optimally and can regulate cells.

Homeostasis within the cell maintains all the numerous functions of the cell at stability, which ensures balance. It may also involve the maintenance of PH, and the saturate concentration levels of the cytoplasm, which is the most significant cell component in terms of volume. All these are aspects of the cell that must stay constant for optimal cell health. Sirtuins perform several functions, among them being the ability to deacetylase proteins called histones. Acetyls are proteins with a physical form of Histones are proteins that contain a condensed form of DNA called chromatins, which prevent the proteins from performing their functions in this acetyl.

The deacetylation, therefore, frees the proteins for the undertaking of their respective functions, given that proteins are the building blocks for the body. Proteins are proverbially referred to as bodybuilding foods. Without Sirtuins, therefore, the bodybuilding foods would fail to build our bodies as they are the critical components for freeing the protein molecules in our cells for their functions.

The Miracle of the Blue Areas

The other evidence for the power of Sirtfoods comes from the 'blue zones.' The blue zones are small regions in the world where people miraculously live longer than everywhere else.

Perhaps most startlingly, you don't just see people live longer in blue zones; you still see them retain energy, vigor, and overall health even in their advanced years. Most of us have a fear of becoming decrepit, immobile, and overall miserable as we age.

Furthermore, we envision this as starting to occur in our forties and fifties while becoming a fixed reality in our sixties, seventies, and eighties. Yet in the blue zones, people live past 100 surprisingly regularly but can walk, work and exercise just as well as those in the younger years. Likewise, they remain mentally slide and don't suffer the cognitive deficits we typically associate with old age.

The blue zones include several areas of the Mediterranean, Japan, Italy and Costa Rica. What do these regions all have in common? They all eat a diet high in Sirt foods. The Mediterranean is famous for its healthy diet involving copious amounts of fish and olive oil. The Japanese savor matcha green tea while the Costa Ricans traditionally indulge in cocoa, coffee and more.

This is the beauty of the Sirt food diet – it isn't trying to make your eating habits artificial and awkward It is merely copying the healthiest practices that already exist around the world.

Sirt Diet and Muscle Mass

In the body, there is a family of genes that function as guardians of our muscles and, when under stress, avoid its breakdown: the sirtuins. SIRT is a potent Muscle Breakdown Inhibitor. As long as SIRT is activated, even when we are fasting, muscle breakdown is prevented, and we continue to burn fat for fuel.

SIRT's benefits aren't ending with preserving muscle mass. The sirtuins work to increase our skeletal muscle mass. We need to delve into the exciting world of stem cells and illustrate how that process functions. Our muscle comprises a particular type of stem cell called a satellite cell that regulates its development and regeneration. Satellite cells just sit there quietly most of the time, but they are activated when a muscle gets damaged or stressed. By things like weight training, this is how our muscles grow stronger. SIRT is essential for activating satellite cells, and without its activity, muscles are significantly smaller because they no longer have the capacity to develop or regenerate properly.[6] However, by increasing SIRT activity, we boost our satellite cells, which encourages muscle growth and recovery.

Sirt Diet and Goodness

There was one aspect we couldn't get our minds around in our pilot study: the people didn't get hungry given a drop-in calorie. In reality, several people struggled to consume all of the food that was offered.

One of the significant advantages of the Sirtfood Diet is that we can achieve significant benefits without the need for a long-term calorie restriction. The very first week of diet is the process of hyper-success, where we pair mild fasting with an excess of strong Sirtfoods for a double blow to weight. So, we predicted sure signs of hunger here, as with all of the fasting regimens. But we've had virtually zero!

We found the answer as we trawled through analysis. It's all thanks to the body's primary appetite-regulating hormone, leptin, called the "satiety hormone." As we feed, leptin decreases, signaling the hypothalamus inhibiting desire to a part of the brain. Conversely, leptin signaling to the mind declines as we fly, which makes us feel thirsty.

Leptin is so effective in controlling appetite that early expectations where it could be treated as a "magic bullet" for combating obesity. But that vision was broken because the metabolic disorder found in obesity causes leptin to avoid correctly functioning. Through obesity, the volume of leptin that can reach the brain is not only decreased, but the hypothalamus also becomes desensitized to its behavior. This is regarded as leptin resistance: there is leptin, but it doesn't work correctly anymore. Therefore, for many overweight individuals, the brain continues to think they are underfed even though they consume plenty, which triggers them to seek calories.

The consequence of this is that while the amount of leptin in the blood is necessary to control appetite, how much of it enters the brain and can affect the hypothalamus is far more relevant. It is here that the Sirtfoods shine.

New evidence indicates that the nutrients present in Sirtfoods have unique advantages in overcoming leptin resistance. This is by increasing leptin delivery to the brain and the hypothalamus' response to leptin behavior.

Going back to our original question: Why doesn't the Sirtfood Diet make people feel hungry? Given a decrease in blood leptin rates during the mild quick, which would usually raise motivation, incorporating Sirtfoods into the diet makes leptin signals more productive, leading to better appetite control. Sirtfoods also has powerful effects on our taste centers, meaning we get a lot more pleasure and satisfaction from our food and therefore don't fall into the overeating trap to feel happy. Sirtuins are expected to be a brand-new concept for even the most committed dietitians. But hitting the sirtuins, our metabolism's master regulators, is the foundation of any effective diet for weight loss. Tragically, the very existence of our modern society, with abundant food and sedentary lifestyles, creates a perfect storm to shut down our sirtuin operation, and we see all around us the effects of this.

The good thing is that we know what sirtuins are, how fat accumulation is managed, and how fat burning is encouraged, and most significantly, how to turn them on. And with this revolutionary breakthrough, the key to successful and lasting weight loss is now yours to bear.

Sirtfood Phases

The plan will detoxify your body for seven days, and then you'll need to keep eating Sirt foods to see the weight coming off, or you'll get it all back. This diet is not very healthy because, for most people, you're eating two of your meals, which isn't sustainable in the long term. It is a diet for those who are following a fantasy and ready to pay for it. It is in no way resembles usual feeding, and I assume it is unhealthy. It is very intense stuff. The green juice revolts and I poured some down the sink. I hated tossing all the harvested fibers onto the compost fire, feeling that I would have enjoyed eating all the juice ingredients in their entire state and that it was better anyway.

Due to the high cost of exotic foods and the amount of time you'll spend juicing and cooking your meals, this diet will be incredibly hard to follow for many reasons. If you don't like matcha or kale, you'll find this diet very hard to follow as many of the Sirtfood Diet recipes contain both of these ingredients. Most people just flat out hated how the drinks smelled and couldn't even bother with the diet. The Sirt Diet program includes two phases:

Phase 1

This process will limit you to 1,000 calories a day for a week and two of your meals will be green drinks rich in Sirtfoods such as lettuce, celery, parsley, green tea and lemon. Even rich in Sirtfoods like beef, chicken, spinach, or buckwheat noodles, you can have one meal per day.

Phase 2

You are permitted to increase the caloric intake to 1,500 calories during this process and you are still consuming the two green drinks. Still, you are now permitted to add another meal to the day, allowing two meals and two beverages. This phase can last up to 14 days. This diet is certainly not for everyone, and it requires a lot of funds and energy to get through the meal preparation. The book includes several recipes about halfway through your reading. Still, many of the ingredients are so unique that consumers found it hard to find them at the grocery store, as well as the tastes were so different in the beginning. Generally, this diet is backed by science, as many case studies have been shown, but the possibility of seeing results from this diet alone is a long shot for the average person.

After The Diet

Those two stages may be repeated as often as you wish for further weight loss.

However, upon finishing those stages, you are advised to start "sirtifying" your diet by consistently integrating sirtfoods into your meals.

There are several Sirtfood Diet books full of creamy recipes. You can also include sirtfoods as a snack in your diet or in recipes that you already have.

You are further encouraged to continue consuming the green juice daily.

Thus, the Sirtfood Diet becomes more of a change in lifestyle than a one-time diet.

Breakfast Recipes

Kale Scramble

Preparation time: 10 minutes

Cooking time: 6 minutes

Servings: 2

Ingredients:

- 4 eggs
- 1/8 teaspoon ground turmeric
- Salt and ground black pepper, to taste
- 1 tablespoon water
- 2 teaspoons olive oil
- 1 cup fresh kale, tough ribs removed and chopped

Directions:

1. In a bowl, add the eggs, turmeric, salt, black pepper, and water, and with a whisk, beat until foamy.
2. In a wok, heat the oil over medium heat.
3. Add the egg mixture and stir to combine.
4. Immediately, reduce the heat to medium-low and cook for about 1–2 minutes, stirring frequently.
5. Stir in the kale and cook for about 3–4 minutes, stirring frequently.
6. Remove from the heat and serve immediately.

Nutrition:

Calories 183

Fat 13.4 g

Carbs 4.3 g

Protein 12.1 g

Buckwheat Porridge

Preparation time: 10 minutes

Cooking time: 15 minutes

Servings: 2

Ingredients:

- 1 cup buckwheat, rinsed
- 1 cup unsweetened almond milk
- 1 cup of water
- 1/2 teaspoon ground cinnamon
- 1/2 teaspoon vanilla extract
- 1–2 tablespoons raw honey
- 1/4 cup fresh blueberries

Directions:

1. In a pan, add all the ingredients (except honey and blueberries) over medium-high heat and bring to a boil.
2. Now, reduce the heat to low and simmer, covered for about 10 minutes.
3. Stir in the honey and remove from the heat.
4. Set aside, covered, for about 5 minutes.
5. With a fork, fluff the mixture and transfer it into serving bowls.
6. Top with blueberries and serve.

Nutrition:

Calories 358

Fat 4.7 g

Carbs 3.7 g

Protein 12 g

Salmon & Kale Omelet

Preparation time: 10 minutes

Cooking time: 7 minutes

Servings: 4

Ingredients:

- 6 eggs
- 2 tablespoons unsweetened almond milk
- Salt and ground black pepper, to taste
- 2 tablespoons olive oil
- 4 ounces smoked salmon, cut into bite-sized chunks
- 2 cup fresh kale, tough ribs removed and chopped finely
- 4 scallions, chopped finely

Directions:

1. In a bowl, place the eggs, coconut milk, salt and black pepper.
2. And beat well.
3. Set aside.
4. In a nonstick wok, heat the oil over medium heat.
5. Place the egg mixture evenly and cook for about 30 seconds, without stirring.
6. Place the salmon, kale and scallions on top of the egg mixture evenly.
7. Now, reduce heat to low.
8. With the lid, cover the wok and cook for about 4–5 minutes.
9. Uncover the wok and cook for about 1 minute.
10. Carefully transfer the omelet onto a serving plate and serve.

Nutrition:

Calories 210

Fat 14.9 g

Carbs 5.2 g

Protein 14.8 g

Moroccan Spiced Eggs

Preparation time: 1 hour

Cooking time: 50 minutes

Servings: 2

Ingredients:

- 1 tsp olive oil
- One shallot, stripped and finely hacked
- One red (chime) pepper, deseeded and finely hacked
- One garlic clove, stripped and finely hacked
- One (zucchini), stripped and finely hacked
- 1 tbsp. tomato puree (glue)
- ½ tsp gentle stew powder
- ¼ tsp ground cinnamon
- ¼ tsp ground cumin
- ½ tsp salt
- 400g (14oz) can hacked tomatoes
- 400g (14oz) may use chickpeas in water
- A little bunch of level leaf parsley (10g (1/3oz)), cleaved
- Four medium eggs at room temperature

Directions:

1. Heat the oil in a pan, include the shallot and red (ringer) pepper, and fry delicately for 5 minutes.
2. At that point, include the garlic and (zucchini) and cook for one more moment or two.
3. Include the tomato puree (glue), flavors, and salt and mix through.
4. Add the cleaved tomatoes and chickpeas (dousing alcohol and all) and increment the warmth to medium.

5. With the top of the dish, stew the sauce for 30 minutes – ensure it is delicately rising all through and permit it to lessen in volume by around 33%.
6. Remove from the warmth and mix in the cleaved parsley.
7. Preheat the grill to 200C/180C fan/350F.

Nutrition:

Calories: 116 kcal

Protein: 6.97 g

Fat: 5.22 g

Carbohydrates: 13.14 g

Chilaquiles with Gochujang

Preparation time: 30 minutes

Cooking time: 20 minutes

Servings: 2

Ingredients:

- One dried ancho chili
- 2 cups of water
- 1 cup squashed tomatoes
- Two cloves of garlic
- One teaspoon genuine salt
- 1/2 tablespoons gochujang
- 5 to 6 cups tortilla chips
- Three enormous eggs
- One tablespoon olive oil

Directions:

1. Get the water to heat a pot.
2. I cheated marginally and heated the water in an electric pot and emptied it into the pan.
3. There's no sound unrivaled strategy here.
4. Add the anchor chili to the bubbled water and drench for 15 minutes to give it an opportunity to stout up.
5. When completed, use tongs or a spoon to extricate chili.
6. Make sure to spare the water for the sauce! Nonetheless, on the off chance that you incidentally dump the water, it's not the apocalypse.
7. Mix the doused chili, 1 cup of saved high temp water, squashed tomatoes, garlic, salt and gochujang until smooth.
8. Empty sauce into a large dish and warmth over medium warmth for 4 to 5 minutes. Mood killer the heat and include the tortilla chips. Mix the chips to cover with the sauce. In a different skillet, shower a teaspoon of oil and fry an egg on top until the whites have settled. Plate the egg and cook the remainder of the eggs. If you are phenomenal at performing various tasks, you can likely sear the eggs while you heat the red sauce. I am not precisely so capable.
9. Top the chips with the seared eggs, cotija, hacked cilantro, jalapeños, onions and avocado. Serve right away.

Nutrition:

Calories: 484 kcal

Protein: 14.55 g

Fat: 18.62 g

Carbohydrates: 64.04 g

Twice Baked Breakfast Potatoes

Preparation time: 1 hour 10 minutes

Cooking time: 1 hour

Servings: 2

Ingredients:

- 2 medium reddish brown potatoes, cleaned and pricked with a fork everywhere
- 2 tablespoons unsalted spread
- 3 tablespoons overwhelming cream
- 4 rashers cooked bacon
- 4 huge eggs
- 1/2 cup destroyed cheddar
- Daintily cut chives
- Salt and pepper to taste

Directions:

1. Preheat grill to 400 degrees F.
2. Spot potatoes straightforwardly on stove rack in the focal point of the grill and prepare for 30 to 45 min.
3. Evacuate and permit potatoes to cool for around 15 minutes.
4. Cut every potato down the middle longwise and burrow every half out, scooping the potato substance into a blending bowl.
5. Gather margarine and cream to the potato and pound into a single unit until smooth — season with salt and pepper and mix.
6. Spread a portion of the potato blend into the base of each emptied potato skin and sprinkle with one tablespoon cheddar (you may make them remain pounded potato left to snack on).
7. Add one rasher bacon to every half and top with a raw egg.
8. Spot potatoes onto a heating sheet and come back to the appliance.
9. Lower broiler temperature to 375 degrees F and heat potatoes until egg whites simply set and yolks are as yet runny.
10. Top every potato with a sprinkle of the rest of the cheddar, season with salt and pepper, and finish with cut chives.

Nutrition:

Calories: 647 kcal

Protein: 30.46 g

Fat: 55.79 g

Carbohydrates: 7.45 g

Sirt Muesli

Preparation time: 30 minutes

Cooking time: 0 minutes

Servings: 2

Ingredients:

- 20g buckwheat drops
- 10g buckwheat puffs
- 15g coconut drops or dried up coconut
- 40g Medjool dates, hollowed and slashed
- 15g pecans, slashed
- 10g cocoa nibs
- 100g strawberries, hulled and slashed
- 100g plain Greek yoghurt (or vegetarian elective, for example, soya or coconut yoghurt)

Directions:

1. Blend the entirety of the above fixings (forget about the strawberries and yoghurt if not serving straight away).

Nutrition:

Calories: 334 kcal

Protein: 4.39 g

Fat: 22.58 g

Carbohydrates: 34.35 g

Mushroom Scramble Eggs

Preparation time: 45 minutes

Cooking time: 10 minutes

Servings: 2

Ingredients:

- 2 eggs
- 1 tsp ground turmeric
- 1 tsp mellow curry powder
- 20g kale, generally slashed
- 1 tsp additional virgin olive oil
- 1/2 superior bean stew, daintily cut
- Bunch of catch mushrooms, meagerly cut
- 5g (3/16oz.) parsley, finely slashed
- *optional* Add a seed blend as a topper and some Rooster Sauce for enhance

Directions:

2. Blend the turmeric and curry powder.
3. Include a little water until you have accomplished a light glue.
4. Steam the kale for 2–3 minutes.
5. Warmth the oil in a skillet over medium heat
6. Fry the bean stew and mushrooms for 2–3 minutes.
7. Include the eggs and flavor glue and cook over a medium warmth at that point.
8. Add the kale and keep on cooking over medium heat for a further moment.
9. At long last, include the parsley, blend well and serve.

Nutrition:

Calories: 158 kcal

Protein: 9.96 g

Fat: 10.93 g

Carbohydrates: 5.04 g

Smoked Salmon Omelets

Preparation time: 45 minutes

Cooking time: 15 minutes

Servings: 2

Ingredients:

- 2 Medium eggs
- 100 g Smoked salmon, cut
- 1/2 tsp Capers
- 10 g Rocket, slashed
- 1 tsp Parsley, slashed
- 1 tsp extra virgin olive oil

Directions:

1. Split the eggs into a bowl and whisk well.
2. Include the salmon, tricks, rocket and parsley.
3. Warmth the olive oil in a nonstick skillet until hot yet not smoking.
4. Include the egg blend and, utilizing a spatula or fish cut, move the mixture around the dish until it is even.
5. Diminish the warmth and let the omelette cook through.
6. Slide the spatula around the edges and move up or crease the omelette fifty-fifty to serve.

Nutrition:

Calories: 148 kcal

Protein: 15.87 g

Fat: 8.73 g

Carbohydrates: 0.36 g

Date and Walnut Porridge

Preparation time: 55 minutes

Cooking time: 30 minutes

Servings: 2

Ingredients:

- 200 ml Milk or without dairy elective
- 1 Medjool date, hacked
- 35 g Buckwheat chips
- 1 tsp. Pecan spread or four cleaved pecan parts
- 50 g Strawberries, hulled

Directions:

1. Spot the milk and time in a dish, heat tenderly, at that point include the buckwheat chips and cook until the porridge is your ideal consistency.
2. Mix in the pecan margarine or pecans, top with the strawberries, and serve.

Nutrition:

Calories: 66 kcal

Protein: 1.08 g

Fat: 1.07 g

Carbohydrates: 14.56 g

Beef Stroganoff French Bread Toast

Preparation time: 10 minutes.

Cooking time: 15 minutes.

Servings: 2.

Ingredients:

- 4 tablespoons olive oil.
- 1/2 cups mushrooms.
- 2 teaspoons salt, separated.
- 1/2 teaspoon dark pepper.
- 2 tablespoons thyme.
- 2 tablespoons spread.
- 1/2 cup onions, diced.
- 2 cloves garlic, minced.
- 1-pound ground meat.
- 3 tablespoons generally useful flour.
- 2 teaspoons paprika.
- 1/2 cups meat juices.
- 1/2 cup sharp cream.
- 1 teaspoon Dijon mustard.
- For the toasts:
- 1 portion French bread, inner parts dugout.
- 2 cups mozzarella.
- 3 tablespoons cleaved Italian parsley.

Directions:

1. Preheat stove to 350 degrees and line a sheet container with material paper.
2. Make the stroganoff:
3. In a large Dutch grill or skillet, heat olive oil over medium warmth.
4. Saute mushrooms with one teaspoon salt and dark pepper. Include thyme. Cook mushrooms until brilliant, roughly 4 minutes.
5. Expel from a dish and put in a safe spot.
6. Include margarine, onions, and garlic to the container and saute 2 minutes.
7. Cook ground hamburger over medium warmth until dark-colored, roughly 4 minutes.
8. Add flour and paprika to cover uniformly.
9. Include meat soup, sour cream, and mustard.
10. Blend entirely and include mushrooms back in round the emptied portion with stroganoff and top with mozzarella cheddar.

11. Spot on the readied heating sheet and prepare for 5 to 10 minutes until cheddar is brilliant and softened.
12. Head with parsley, cut and serve right away.

Nutrition:

Calories: 1007 kcal.

Protein: 88.04 g.

Fat: 60 g.

Carbohydrates: 32.06 g.

Classic French Toast

Preparation time: 10 minutes.

Cooking time: 45 minutes.

Servings: 2.

Ingredients:

- Four huge eggs.
- 1/2 cup whole milk.
- One teaspoon vanilla concentrate.
- 1/2 teaspoons ground cinnamon partitioned.
- 8 cuts Brioche bread.

Directions:

1. On the off chance that is utilizing an electric iron, preheat the frying pan to 350°F.
2. Race until very much consolidated.
3. Plunge each side of the bread in the egg blend.
4. Note - include the other portion of the cinnamon after you have plunged half of your bread cuts and blend once more.
5. This will ensure the entirety of the cuts gets a decent measure of cinnamon.
6. Soften a little margarine on the hot frying pan or in a large skillet over medium warmth.

7. Serve the French toast warm with maple syrup, powdered sugar and berries, whenever wanted.
8. Note - to keeps the French toast warm, heat the stove to 200°F. Spot a wire rack on a massive preparing sheet and spot the French toast on the shelf. Keep warm in the grill for as long as 30 minutes.

Nutrition:

Calories: 110.

Fat: 11g.

Carbs: 26.5g.

Protein: 2.5g.

Avocado and Kale Omelet

Preparation time: 10 minutes.

Cooking time: 45 minutes.

Servings: 2.

Ingredients:

- Two enormous eggs.
- One teaspoon low-fat milk.
- Spot of salt.
- Two teaspoons extra-virgin olive oil, partitioned.
- 1 cup cleaved kale.
- One tablespoon lime juice.
- One tablespoon cleaved fresh cilantro.
- One teaspoon unsalted sunflower seed.
- Spot of squashed red pepper.
- Spot of salt.
- ¼ avocado, cut.

Directions:

1. Mix eggs with milk and salt in a little bowl.
2. Warmth 1 teaspoon oil in a little nonstick skillet over medium warmth.
3. Include the egg blend and cook until the base is set and the inside is still somewhat runny 1 to 2 minutes.
4. Flip the omelet over and cook until set, around 30 seconds more. Move to a plate.
5. Hurl kale with the staying one teaspoon oil, lime juice, cilantro, sunflower seeds, squashed red pepper and a touch of salt.
6. Top the omelet with the kale plate of mixed greens and avocado.

Nutrition:

Calories: 339.

Fat: 28.1g.

Carbs: 13g.

Protein: 15g.

Easy Egg-White Muffins

Preparation time: 10 minutes.

Cooking time: 15 minutes.

Servings: 2.

Ingredients:

- English muffin.
- Egg-whites - 6 tbsp. or two large egg whites.
- Turkey bacon or bacon sausage.
- Sharp cheddar cheese or gouda.
- Organic berry.
- Optional – lettuce and hot sauce, hummus, flaxseeds, etc...

Directions:

1. Get a microwavable safe container, then spray entirely to stop the egg from adhering, then pour egg whites into the dish.
2. Lay turkey bacon or bacon sausage paper towel and then cook.
3. Subsequently, toast your muffin, if preferred.
4. Then put the egg dish in the microwave for 30 minutes.
5. Afterward, with a spoon or fork, then immediately flip egg within the dish and cook for another 30 minutes.
6. Whilst the dish remains hot, sprinkle some cheese while preparing sausage.
7. The secret is to get a paste of some kind between each coating to put up the sandwich together, i.e. - a very small little bit of hummus or even cheese.

Nutrition:

Calories: 371.

Fat: 22g.

Carbs: 25g.

Protein: 23g.

Avocado Eggs with Toast

Preparation time: 10 minutes.

Cooking time: 45 minutes.

Servings: 2.

Ingredients:

- One avocado.
- 4 cuts whole wheat sandwich bread.
- Two tablespoons avocado oil.
- Four medium eggs.
- ¼ teaspoon salt, separated.
- ¼ teaspoon ground pepper, separated.
- Four tablespoons salsa.

Directions:

1. Preheat stove to 375°F. Coat a huge rimmed preparing sheet with cooking splash.
2. Split avocado and strip.
3. Cut the long way into 1/4-inch-thick cuts, so you have cut through the entire length of the avocado with the gap from the pit.
4. Separate the four cuts nearest to either side of the hole and the shallow cuts; put in a safe spot.
5. Utilizing a baked good brush, delicately cover the two sides of each cut of bread with oil.
6. Cut a piece out of the focal point of each bread cut, looking like an avocado cut.
7. Move the dough and slice out bread pieces to the readied heating sheet.
8. Spot the shallow avocado cuts in the gaps of the bread.
9. Split an egg over every one of the avocado cuts in the dough.
10. Sprinkle the eggs with 1/8 teaspoon salt and 1/8 teaspoon pepper.
11. Each egg with one of the avocado cuts taken from the part nearest to the pit with an opening in them, uncovering the egg.
12. Sprinkle the avocado with the staying 1/8 teaspoon salt and 1/8 teaspoon pepper.
13. Prepare until the toast has seared in spots and the eggs are simply set 10 to 12 minutes.
14. Top with salsa, whenever wanted.
15. Present with the cut-out bread pieces.

Nutrition: 285 calories; 20.1 g absolute fat; 3.6 g-soaked fat; 186 mg cholesterol; 347 mg sodium. 386 mg potassium; 10.8 g protein.

Baked Oatmeal

Preparation time: 10 minutes.

Cooking time: 25 minutes.

Servings: 2.

Ingredients:

- 2 cups old-fashioned oats.
- ½ cup pecans, hacked.
- Two teaspoons ground cinnamon.
- One teaspoon preparing powder.
- ¾ teaspoon salt.
- 1/4 teaspoon ground nutmeg.
- 1/8 teaspoon ground cloves.
- 2 cups unsweetened almond milk or 2% milk.
- 1 cup low-fat plain Greek yoghurt.
- ¼ cup pure maple syrup.
- Two tablespoons extra-virgin olive oil.
- One teaspoon vanilla concentrate.
- Two pears diced little.
- 1/3 Cup low-fat plain Greek yoghurt.

Directions:

1. Preheat stove to 375°F. Coat a 9-inch-square preparing dish with cooking shower.
2. Blend oats, pecans, cinnamon, heating powder, salt, nutmeg and cloves in an enormous bowl.
3. Whisk almond milk (or milk), 1 cup yoghurt, maple syrup, oil and vanilla in a medium bowl.
4. Empty the wet fixings into the dry fixings.
5. Delicately blend in.
6. Move the blend to the readied heating dish.
7. Heat until brilliant darker, 45 to 55 minutes.

Nutrition:

Calories: 311.

Fat: 14.8g.

Carbs: 12.1g.

Protein: 9.3g.

Sirt cereal

Preparation time: 15 minutes

Cooking time: 1 hour 20 minutes

Servings: 2-3

Ingredients:

- 50 g coconut oil
- 150 ml clear honey
- 1 tbsp ground turmeric
- 100 goats (use certified gluten-free oats if you're avoiding gluten)
- 250 g buckwheat flakes
- 100 g walnuts, chopped
- 50 g pecans, chopped
- 50 g flaked almonds
- 30 g pumpkin seeds
- 30 g sunflower seeds and 50 g cocoa nibs

Directions:

1. Heat your oven to 160 ° C / gas 3.
2. In a small saucepan, melt the coconut oil and honey over low heat and then stir in the turmeric.
3. Mix well to make sure no lumps are formed.
4. Mix all dry ingredients in a bowl and stir in the oil and honey.
5. Make sure they combine well then transfer them to a nonstick baking sheet or one lined with parchment paper.
6. Bake for 35–40 minutes, stirring for half the cooking time.
7. Once it's a nice golden color, remove it and let it cool on the baking sheet

before storing in an airtight container for up to two months.

Nutrition:

Carbohydrates: 28 | Fat: 7 | Protein: 6 | Kcal: 220

Sirt breakfast bar

Preparation time: 15 minutes

Cooking time: approx. 2 hours

Servings: 10

Ingredients:

- 150 g pitted Medjool dates, chopped
- 150 g walnut butter
- 50 g thick honey
- 375 g sirtfood muesli

Directions:

1. Put the dates, walnut butter and honey in a food processor and blend until you have a nice paste. This can take some time as the dates won't be crushed and you will have to scrape the sides of the bowl a few times. Transfer the paste to a mixing bowl and stir the granola, making sure it is well mixed. If you squeeze a lump of the mixture in your hand, it should stay firm.
2. Line a 25 × 18 cm baking pan with parchment paper and spoon the mixture into it. Use your hands or the back of a spoon to spread it around the can as evenly as possible, then blot firmly to make sure the bars stay in one piece as you cut. Alternatively, you can shape the mixture into bite-sized balls.
3. Chill at least 2 hours before attempting to cut the mixture into about 10 bars. You can then store them in an airtight

container in the refrigerator for up to two weeks.

Nutrition:

Carbohydrates: 23 | Fat: 5 | Protein: 3 | Kcal: 140

Sirt cocoa pops

Preparation time: 10 minutes

Cooking time: 25 minutes

Servings: 10

Ingredients:

- 100 g corn
- 1 extra virgin olive oil or melted coconut oil
- For covering
- 50 g walnuts, chopped
- 50 g sunflower seeds
- 50 g buckwheat flakes
- 35 g cocoa nibs
- For serving
- 1 teaspoon cocoa powder (100 percent)
- 1 Medjool date, finely chopped
- 200 ml milk or dairy-free alternative

Directions:

1. Heat the oven to 160 ° C / gas 3.
2. Place a heavy pan with a tightly fitting lid over medium heat.
3. Mix the corn and oil, pour the mixture into the hot pan and cover with the lid.
4. Shake the pan to get the corn moving in it.
5. Once it starts to pop, turn up the heat and shake the pan for as long as you can while the lid is still on.
6. Once the popping has settled down to about 2 to 3 seconds between pops,

remove the pan from the heat and empty it into a bowl.
7. Discard any kernels that have not popped, allow to cool completely, then transfer to an airtight container and store for up to a week.
8. For the topping, place the walnuts and sunflower seeds in a small baking sheet and roast in the oven for 15 minutes. Transfer to a bowl and mix with the buckwheat and cocoa nibs.
9. Let it cool completely and then store it in an airtight container for up to 1 month. The corn and topping should be stored separately to ensure even distribution when serving.
10. To serve, add 1–2 tablespoons of toppings and 10 g of popcorn to a bowl. Stir the cocoa powder and date into the milk then pour it over the grain.

Nutrition:

Carbohydrates: 21 | Fat: 14 | Protein: 3 | Kcal: 230

Sirt fruit bowl

Preparation time: 15 minutes

Cooking time: 0 minutes

Servings: 1

Ingredients:

- 40 g (10) raspberries
- 60 g (10) red / black grapes, halved
- 80 g (1 medium) plum, chopped
- 60 g (½ medium)
- Apple, cut
- 50 g (2 medium) peeled strawberries, chopped
- Juice of ¼ lemon
- 100 g Greek yogurt
- 5 walnut halves, mashed

Directions:

1. Put all the fruits in a bowl. Squeeze the lemon juice over it and mix well.
2. Pour over the Greek yogurt, sprinkle the chopped walnuts on top, and serve.

Nutrition:

Carbohydrates: 24 | Fat: 17 | Protein: 3 | Kcal: 180

Grilled sausages with fried Onions and scrambled eggs with herbs

Preparation time: 10 minutes

Cooking time: 20 minutes

Servings: 1

Ingredients:

- 2 lean pork or beef sausages 2 eggs
- 1 teaspoon chopped parsley
- 1 teaspoon chopped chives
- 25 ml milk or dairy-free alternative
- 1 teaspoon extra virgin olive oil
- 60 g red onion
- 1 teaspoon dried thyme

Directions:

1. Heat a grill on the highest setting.
2. Grill the sausages for 8 to 10 minutes, turning them from time to time until they are browned nicely all over.
3. Whisk eggs, parsley, chives and milk together.
4. Put ½ teaspoon of olive oil in a small saucepan over medium heat, add the egg mixture and cook gently until you have a nice scrambled egg.
5. In the meantime, put the remaining ½ teaspoon of olive oil in a small pan over medium heat and fry the onion and thyme for 3-4 minutes until brown.
6. Stack the eggs on a plate and cover with the sausages and onions.

Nutrition:

Carbohydrates: 24 | Fat: 27 | Protein: 15 | Kcal: 420

Smoked salmon, arugula and Capers on buckwheat crackers

Preparation time: 10 minutes

Cooking time: 15 minutes

Servings: 1

Ingredients:

- 1 teaspoon capers
- 60 g Greek yogurt
- 1 tbsp. chopped parsley
- 10 g red onion, thinly sliced
- Buckwheat crackers
- 75 g smoked salmon
- 20 g rocket juice from ¼ lemon

Directions:

1. Mix capers, yoghurt, parsley and onion in a bowl.
2. Spread the mixture over your crackers and top with the smoked salmon and arugula.
3. Finally, squeeze out some lemon juice.

Nutrition:

Carbohydrates: 15 | Fat: 7 | Protein: 3 | Kcal: 120

Baked Kipper with Kale and poached eggs

Preparation time: 10 minutes

Cooking time: 20 minutes

Servings: 1

Ingredients:

- 1 tipper 1 tsp
- extra virgin olive oil
- 1 teaspoon chopped parsley
- 50 g kale, chopped
- A few drops of vinegar
- 1 medium egg
- 1 lemon wedge

Directions:

1. Preheat your oven to 200 ° C / gas 6.
2. In the meantime, bring 2 small pots of water to a boil.
3. If necessary, cut the head and tail off your kipper
4. Place the skin-side down on a piece of foil.
5. Pour the olive oil and parsley over the kipper and wrap the foil around it.
6. Place the kale in a pan of boiling water and simmer for 5 minutes or until tender.
7. Drain and keep warm.
8. Put a few drops of vinegar in the other pan with boiling water.
9. and let the heat simmer.
10. Stir the water clockwise and then crack your egg in half.
11. An egg with a solid white and liquid yolk takes 2 to 3 minutes.
12. Remove with a slotted spoon and drain on kitchen paper.
13. Serve the egg on top of the kipper with the kale aside.

Nutrition:

Carbohydrates: 11 | Fat: 17 | Protein: 33 | Kcal: 340

Poached egg with rocket, Asparagus and bacon

Preparation time: 5 minutes

Cooking time: 15 minutes

Servings: 1

Ingredients:

- 2 slices of striped or bacon back
- 6 asparagus spears,
- a few drops of vinegar 2 eggs
- 10 g rocket
- 1 teaspoon extra virgin olive oil

Directions:

1. Heat a grill on the highest setting.
2. In the meantime, bring 2 small pots of water to the boil.
3. Once the grill is hot, grill your bacon until the fat is crispy.
4. Put the asparagus spears in a pan of boiling water.
5. And cook for 2-3 minutes until tender.
6. Put a few drops of vinegar in the other pan with boiling water.
7. And let the heat simmer.
8. Stir the water clockwise and then crack an egg in the middle.
9. An egg with a solid white and liquid yolk takes 2 to 3 minutes.
10. Remove with a slotted spoon and drain on kitchen paper.
11. Cook the second egg in the same way.
12. Place the eggs on the asparagus.
13. Cover with the crispy bacon and rocket and drizzle over the olive oil.

Nutrition:

Carbohydrates: 11 | Fat: 17 | Protein: 33 | Kcal: 340

Strawberry and Cherry Smoothie

Preparation time: 5 minutes

Cooking time: 0 minutes

Servings: 1

Ingredients:

- 100g (3½ oz.) strawberries
- 75g (3oz) frozen pitted cherries
- 1 tablespoon plain full-fat yogurt
- 175mls (6fl oz.) unsweetened soya milk
- Serves 1
- 132 calories per serving

Directions:

1. Place all of the ingredients into a blender and process until smooth.
2. Serve and enjoy.

Eggs with Kale

Preparation time: 5 minutes

Cooking time: 10 minutes

Servings: 1

Ingredients:

- 2 large eggs
- Salt
- Ground black pepper
- 1 tsp. olive oil or avocado oil
- 1 cup kale

Directions:

1. Heat 1 tsp. olive oil in the skillet over (medium/high) heat.
2. Add kale and cook, tossing, until wilted (Approx. 1 minute).
3. Remove kale, add eggs and fry until done.
4. Serve with kale.

Banana Snap

Preparation time: 5 minutes

Cooking time: 0 minutes

Servings: 1

Ingredients:

- 2.5cm (1 inch) chunk of fresh ginger, peeled
- 1 banana
- 1 large carrot
- 1 apple, cored
- ½ stick of celery
- ¼ level teaspoon turmeric powder

Directions:

1. Place all the ingredients into a blender with just enough water to cover them.
2. Process until smooth
3. Nutrients: 166 calories per serving

Green Egg Scramble

Preparation time: 5 minutes

Cooking time: 10 minutes

Servings: 1

Ingredients:

- 2 eggs, whisked
- 25g (1oz) rocket (arugula) leaves
- 1 teaspoon chives, chopped
- 1 teaspoon fresh basil, chopped
- 1 teaspoon fresh parsley, chopped
- 1 tablespoon olive oil

Directions:

1. Mix the eggs together with the rocket (arugula) and herbs.
2. Heat the oil in a frying pan and pour into the egg mixture.
3. Gently stir until it's lightly scrambled.

4. Season and serve.

Nutrients: 250 calories

Strawberry Blend

Preparation time: 5 minutes + 8h

Cooking time: 0 minutes

Servings: 2

Ingredients:

- 2 oz. rolled oats
- 4 oz. almond milk, unsweetened
- 2 tbsp. plain yoghurt
- 1 cup strawberries
- 1 tsp honey
- 1 square 85% chocolate

Directions:

1. Mix the oats and the milk and leave overnight.
2. In the morning top the jar with yoghurt, honey, strawberries and chocolate.
3. Cut in small pieces.

Nutrition:

Calories: 258, Fat: 3.3g, Carbohydrate: 29.8g, Protein: 13.6g

Avocado Kale smoothie

Preparation time: 5 minutes

Cooking time: 10 minutes

Servings: 1

Ingredients:

- 3 stalks of kales
- 1 avocado, peeled & de-stoned
- 1 teaspoon fresh parsley
- ½ teaspoon matcha powder
- Juice of ½ lemon

Directions:

1. Place all of the ingredients into a blender and add enough water to cover them.
2. Process until creamy and smooth.

Nutrition: 306 calories

Green Sirtfood Smoothie

Preparation time: 5 minutes

Cooking time: 0 minutes

Servings: 1

Ingredients:

- 100g unsweetened Greek yoghurt
- 6 walnut halves
- 8-10 medium strawberries
- a handful of kale leaves
- 20g dark chocolate (min. 85% cocoa)
- 1 date
- 1/2 teaspoon turmeric
- Small piece fresh chili, finely chopped
- 200ml unsweetened almond milk

Directions:

1. Put everything into a blender and mix until you get a smoothie.

Nutrition: 250 calories

Power cereals

Preparation time: 5 minutes

Cooking time: 5 minutes

Servings: 1

For one serving. The ultimate start to the day with extra sirtuin foods.

- 20g buckwheat flakes
- 10g puffed buckwheat
- 15g coconut flakes
- 40g Medjool dates, seeded and chopped
- 10g cocoa nibs
- 100g strawberries
- 100g Greek natural yoghurt

Directions:

1. Mix all ingredients together.
2. If you are preparing on stock, e.g. for five portions, simply take five times the amount.
3. You can store them for a few days in an airtight tin.
4. If you prefer to eat vegan, use soy yoghurt instead of Greek yoghurt.
5. Instead of strawberries you can also use other berries, e.g. raspberries, blueberries or blackberries.

Nutrition: 350 calories

Berry Yoghurt

Preparation time: 5 minutes

Cooking time: 0 minutes

Servings: 1

For breakfast as part of your sirtfood diet we suggest this yoghurt for example:

Ingredients:

- 125g mixed berries, e.g. blueberries, strawberries and blackberries
- 150g Greek yoghurt
- 25g walnuts, chopped
- 10g dark chocolate (85%), grated

Directions:

1. Simply mix all ingredients together.
2. Vegans can also use soy yoghurt and vegan chocolate instead of yoghurt.

Nutrition: 250 calories

Yoghurt with berries

Preparation time: 5 minutes

Cooking time: 0 minutes

Servings: 1

Ingredients:

- Unsweetened yoghurt (125g)
- Fresh berries, e.g. raspberries, approx. 60g.

Directions:

1. Mix all ingredients

Nutrition: 150 calories

Raspberries belong to the so-called Sirt foods - and so this breakfast is also suitable as part of a Sirt food diet.

Blueberry frozen yogurt

Preparation time: 5 minutes

Cooking time: 0 minutes

Servings: 4

Ingredients:

- 450g (1lb) plain yogurt
- 175g (6oz) blueberries
- Juice of 1 orange
- 1 tablespoon honey

Directions:

1. Place the blueberries and orange juice into a food processor or blender and blitz until smooth. Press the mixture

through a sieve into a large bowl to remove seeds. Stir in the honey and yogurt. Transfer the mixture to an ice-cream maker and follow the manufacturer's instructions. Alternatively pour the mixture into a container and place in the fridge for 1 hour. Use a fork to whisk it and break up ice crystals and freeze for 2 hours.

Nutrition: 133 calories per serving

Vegetable & Nut Loaf

Preparation time: 5 minutes

Cooking time: 0 minutes

Servings: 4

Ingredients:

- 175g (6oz) mushrooms, finely chopped
- 100g (3½ oz) haricot beans
- 100g (3½ oz) walnuts, finely chopped
- 100g (3½ oz) peanuts, finely chopped
- 1 carrot, finely chopped
- 3 sticks celery, finely chopped
- 1 bird's-eye chilli, finely chopped
- 1 red onion, finely chopped
- 1 egg, beaten
- 2 cloves of garlic, chopped
- 2 tablespoons olive oil
- 2 teaspoons turmeric powder
- 2 tablespoons soy sauce
- 4 tablespoons fresh parsley, chopped
- 100mls (3½ fl. oz.) water
- 60mls (2fl oz.) red wine

Directions:

1. Heat the oil in a pan.
2. Add the garlic, chili, carrot, celery, onion, mushrooms and turmeric.
3. Cook for 5 minutes.

4. Grease and line a large loaf tin with greaseproof paper.
5. Let it stand for 10 minutes then turn onto a serving plate.

Nutrition: 453 calories per serving

Dates & Parma Ham

Preparation time: 5 minutes

Cooking time: 0 minutes

Servings: 1

Ingredients:

- 12 medjool dates
- 2 slices of Parma ham, cut into strips
- Serves 4
- 202 calories per serving

Directions:

1. Wrap each date with a strip of Parma ham.
2. Can be served hot or cold.

Nutrition: 250 calories

Braised Celery

Preparation time: 5 minutes

Cooking time: 0 minutes

Servings: 1

Ingredients:

- 250g (9oz) celery, chopped
- 100mls (3½ fl oz) warm vegetable stock (broth)
- 1 red onion, chopped
- 1 clove of garlic, crushed
- 1 tablespoon fresh parsley, chopped
- 25g (1oz) butter

- Sea salt and freshly ground black pepper

Directions:

1. Place the celery, onion, stock (broth) and garlic into a saucepan simmer for 10 minutes.
2. Stir in the parsley and butter and season with salt and pepper.
3. Serve as an accompaniment to roast meat dishes.

Nutrition: 67 calories

Cheesy Buckwheat Cakes

Preparation time: 5 minutes

Cooking time: 0 minutes

Servings: 1

Ingredients:

- 100g (3½oz) buckwheat, cooked and cooled
- 1 large egg
- 25g (1oz) cheddar cheese, grated (shredded)
- 25g (1oz) whole meal breadcrumbs
- 2 shallots, chopped
- 2 tablespoons fresh parsley, chopped
- 1 tablespoon olive oil

Directions:

1. Crack the egg into a bowl, whisk it then set aside.
2. In a separate bowl combine all the buckwheat, cheese, shallots and parsley.
3. Mix well.
4. Pour in the beaten egg to the buckwheat mixture and stir well.
5. Shape the mixture into patties.

6. Scatter the breadcrumbs on a plate and roll the patties in them.
7. Heat the olive oil in a large frying pan.
8. And gently place the cakes in the oil.
9. Cook for 3-4 minutes on either side until slightly golden.

Nutrition: 358 calories

Red Chicory & Stilton Cheese Boats

Preparation time: 5 minutes

Cooking time: 0 minutes

Servings: 1

Ingredients:

- 200g (7oz) stilton cheese, crumbled
- 200g (7oz) red chicory leaves (or if unavailable, use yellow)
- 2 tablespoon fresh parsley, chopped
- 1 tablespoon olive oil

Directions:

1. Place the red chicory leaves onto a baking sheet.
2. Drizzle them with olive oil then sprinkle the cheese inside the leaves.
3. Place them under a hot grill (broiler) for around 4 minutes.
4. Sprinkle with chopped parsley and serve straight away.

Nutrition: 250 calories

Green Omelette

Preparation time: 10 min

Cooking time: 5 min

Servings: 1

Ingredients:

- 2 large eggs, at room temperature
- 1 shallot, peeled and chopped
- Handful arugula
- 3 sprigs of parsley, chopped
- 1 tsp. extra virgin olive oil
- Salt and black pepper

Directions:

1. Beat the eggs in a small bowl and set aside; sauté the shallot for 5 minutes with a bit of the oil, on low-medium heat.
2. Pour the eggs in the pans, stirring the mixture for just a second.
3. The eggs on a medium heat and tip the pan just enough to let the loose egg run underneath after about one minute on the burner.
4. Add the greens, herbs and the seasonings to the top side as it is still soft.
5. TIP: You do not even have to flip it, as you can just cook the egg slowly egg as is well (being careful as not to burn).
6. TIP: Another option is to put it into an oven to broil for 3-5 minutes (checking to make sure it is only until it is golden but burned).

Nutrition: 234 calories

Berry Oat Breakfast Cobbler

Preparation time: 40 min

Cooking time: 5 min

Servings: 2

Ingredients:

- 2 cups of oats/flakes that are ready without cooking
- 1 cup of blackcurrants without the stems

- 1 teaspoon of honey (or ¼ teaspoon of raw sugar)
- ½ cup of water (add more or less by testing the pan)
- 1 cup of plain yogurt (or soy or coconut)

Directions:

1. Boil the berries, honey, and water, and then turn it down on low.
2. Put in a glass container in a refrigerator until it is cool and set (about 30 minutes or more)
3. When ready to eat, scoop the berries on top of the oats and yogurt.
4. Serve immediately.

Nutrition: 241 calories

Pancakes with Apples and Blackcurrants

Preparation time: 30 min

Cooking time: 10 min

Servings: 4

Ingredients:

- 2 apples, cut into small chunks
- 2 cups of quick cooking oats
- 1 cup flour of your choice
- 1 tsp. baking powder
- 2 tbsp. Raw sugar, coconut sugar, or 2 tbsp. honey that is warm and easy to distribute
- 2 egg whites
- 1 ¼ cups of milk (or soy/rice/coconut)
- 2 tsp. extra virgin olive oil
- A dash of salt
- For the berry topping:
- 1 cup blackcurrants, washed and stalks removed

- 3 tbsp. water (may use less)
- 2 tbsp. sugar (see above for types)

Directions:

1. Place the ingredients for the topping in a small pot simmer, stirring frequently for about 10 minutes until it cooks down and the juices are released.
2. Take the dry ingredients and mix in a bowl.
3. After, add the apples and the milk a bit at a time (you may not use it all), until it is a batter.
4. Stiffly whisk the egg whites and then gently mix them into the pancake batter.
5. Set aside in the refrigerator.
6. Pour a one quarter of the oil onto a flat pan or flat griddle and when hot, pour some of the batter into it in a pancake shape.
7. When the pancakes start to have golden brown edges and form air bubbles, they may be ready to be gently flipped.
8. Test to be sure the bottom can life away from the pan before actually flipping.
9. Repeat for the three pancakes.
10. Top each pancake with the berries.

Nutrition: 337 calories

Granola- The Sirt Way

Preparation time: 30 min

Cooking time: 0 min

Servings: 1

Ingredients:

- 1 cup buckwheat puffs
- 1 cup buckwheat flakes (ready to eat type, but not whole buckwheat that needs to be cooked) ½ cup coconut flakes
- ½ cup Medjool dates, without pits, chopped into smaller, bite-sized pieces
- 1 cup of cacao nibs or very dark chocolate chips
- 1/2 cup walnuts, chopped
- 1 cup strawberries chopped and without stem 1 cup plain Greek, or coconut or soy yogurt.

Directions:

1. Mix, without yogurt and strawberry toppings
2. You can store for up to a week, store in an airtight container.
3. Add toppings (even different berries or different yogurt.
4. You can even use the berry toppings as you will learn how to make from other recipes.

Nutrition: 235 Cal

Summer Berry Smoothie

Preparation time: 30 min

Cooking time: 0 min

Servings: 1

Ingredients:

- 50g (2oz) blueberries
- 50g (2oz) strawberries
- 25g (1oz) blackcurrants
- 25g (1oz) red grapes
- 1 carrot, peeled
- 1 orange, peeled
- Juice of 1 lime

Directions:

1. Place all of the ingredients into a blender and cover them with water.
2. Blitz until smooth.
3. You can also add some crushed ice and a mint leaf to garnish.

Nutrition: 300 Cal

Mango, Celery & Ginger Smoothie

Preparation time: 30 min

Cooking time: 0 min

Servings: 1

Ingredients:

- 1 stalk of celery
- 50g (2oz) kale
- 1 apple, cored
- 50g (2oz) mango, peeled, de-stoned and chopped
- 2.5cm (1 inch) chunk of fresh ginger root, peeled and chopped

Directions:

1. Put all the ingredients into a blender with some water and blitz until smooth.
2. Add ice to make your smoothie really refreshing.

Nutrition: 275 Cal

Orange, Carrot & Kale Smoothie

Preparation time: 30 min

Cooking time: 0 min

Servings: 1

Ingredients:

- 1 carrot, peeled
- 1 orange, peeled
- 1 stick of celery

- 1 apple, cored
- 50g (2oz) kale
- ½ teaspoon Matcha powder

Directions:

1. Place all of the ingredients into a blender and add in enough water to cover them.
2. Process until smooth, serve and enjoy.

Nutrition: 279 Cal

Creamy Strawberry & Cherry Smoothie

Preparation time: 30 min

Cooking time: 0 min

Servings: 1

Ingredients:

- 100g (3½ oz.) strawberries
- 75g (3oz) frozen pitted cherries
- 1 tablespoon plain full-fat yogurt
- 175mls (6fl oz.) unsweetened soya milk

Directions:

1. Place all of the ingredients into a blender and process until smooth.
2. Serve and enjoy.

Nutrition: 280 Cal

Grape, Celery & Parsley Reviver

Preparation time: 30 min

Cooking time: 0 min

Servings: 1

Ingredients:

- 75g (3oz) red grapes

- 3 sticks of celery
- 1 avocado, de-stoned and peeled
- 1 tablespoon fresh parsley
- ½ teaspoon Matcha powder

Directions:

1. Place all of the ingredients into a blender with enough water to cover them.
2. And blitz until smooth and creamy.
3. Add crushed ice to make it even more refreshing.

Nutrition: 230Cal

STrawberry & Citrus Blend

Preparation time: 30 min

Cooking time: 0 min

Servings: 1

Ingredients:

- 75g (3oz) strawberries
- 1 apple, cored
- 1 orange, peeled
- ½ avocado, peeled and de-stoned
- ½ teaspoon Matcha powder
- Juice of 1 lime

Directions:

1. Place all of the ingredients into a blender with enough water to cover them.
2. And process until smooth.

Nutrition: 250 Cal

Grapefruit & Celery Blast

Preparation time: 30 min

Cooking time: 0 min

Servings: 1

Ingredients:

- 1 grapefruit, peeled
- 2 stalks of celery
- 50g (2oz) kale
- ½ teaspoon Matcha powder

Directions:

1. Place all the ingredients into a blender with enough water to cover them.
2. Blitz until smooth.

Nutrition: 286 Cal

Orange & Celery Crush

Preparation time: 30 min

Cooking time: 0 min

Servings: 1

Ingredients:

- 1 carrot, peeled
- 3 stalks of celery
- 1 orange, peeled
- ½ teaspoon Matcha powder
- Juice of 1 lime

Directions:

1. Place all of the ingredients into a blender with enough water to cover them.
2. Blitz until smooth.

Nutrition: 274 Cal

Tropical Chocolate Delight

Preparation time: 30 min

Cooking time: 0 min

Servings: 1

Ingredients:

- 1 mango, peeled & de-stoned
- 75g (3oz) fresh pineapple, chopped
- 50g (2oz) kale
- 25g (1oz) rocket
- 1 tablespoon 100% cocoa powder or cacao nibs
- 150mls (5fl oz.) coconut milk

Directions:

1. Place all of the ingredients into a blender and blitz until smooth.
2. You can add a little water if it seems too thick.

Nutrition: 288 Cal

Walnut & Spiced Apple Tonic

Preparation time: 30 min

Cooking time: 0 min

Servings: 1

Ingredients:

- 6 walnuts halves
- 1 apple, cored
- 1 banana
- ½ teaspoon Matcha powder
- ½ teaspoon cinnamon
- Pinch of ground nutmeg

Directions:

1. Place all of the ingredients into a blender and add sufficient water to cover them.
2. Blitz until smooth and creamy.

Nutrition: 258 Cal

Pineapple & Cucumber Smoothie

Preparation time: 30 min

Cooking time: 0 min

Servings: 1

Ingredients:

- 50g (2oz) cucumber
- 1 stalk of celery
- 2 slices of fresh pineapple
- 2 sprigs of parsley
- ½ teaspoon Matcha powder
- A squeeze of lemon juice

Directions:

1. Place all of the ingredients into a blender with enough water to cover them.
2. Blitz until smooth.

Nutrition: 260 Cal

Kale & Orange Juice

Preparation time: 10 minutes

Cooking time: 0 minutes

Servings: 2

Ingredients:

- 5 large oranges, peeled
- 2 bunches fresh kale

Directions:

1. Add all ingredients into a juicer
2. And extract the juice according to the manufacturers.
3. Pour into 2 glasses and serve immediately.

Nutrition: 258 Cal

Orange Juice

Preparation time: 10 minutes

Cooking time: 0 minutes

Servings: 2

Ingredients:

- 5 large oranges, peeled and portioned
- 2 bunches fresh kale

Directions:

1. Add all ingredients into a juicer and extract the juice according to the manufacturer's method.
2. Pour into 2 glasses and serve immediately.

Nutrition: 258 Cal

Apple & Cucumber Juice

Preparation time: 10 minutes

Cooking time: 0 minutes

Servings: 2

Ingredients:

- 3 large apples, cored and sliced
- 2 large cucumbers, sliced
- 4 celery stalks
- 1 (1-inch) piece fresh ginger, peeled
- 1 lemon, peeled

Directions:

1. Add all ingredients into a juicer
2. And extract the juice according to the manufacturer's method.
3. Pour into 2 glasses and serve immediately.

Nutrition: 258 Cal

Hot chorizo, tomato & kale salad

Preparation time: 5 Minutes

Cooking Time: 20 Minutes

Servings: 4

Ingredients:

- 225g (8oz) kale leaves, finely chopped
  75g (3oz) chorizo sausage, thinly sliced
  8 cherry tomatoes
- 2 cloves of garlic
- 1 red onion, finely chopped
- 2 tablespoons olive oil
- 2 tablespoons red wine vinegar sea salt
- Freshly ground black pepper

Directions:

1. Heat the olive oil into a frying pan and add the sliced chorizo, garlic, onion and tomatoes. Cook for around 5 minutes. Add in the red wine vinegar and kale and cook for around 7 minutes or until the kale has softened. Season with salt and pepper. Serve immediately.

Nutrition: 355 calories per serving

Red chicory & walnut coleslaw

Preparation time: 5 Minutes

Cooking Time: 45 Minutes

Servings: 4

Ingredients:

- 100g (3½ oz.) red chicory, (or yellow) finely grated (shredded) 5 stalks of celery, finely chopped 8 walnut halves, chopped
- 1 red onion, finely chopped
- 2 tablespoons mayonnaise

Directions:

1. Place all of the ingredients into a bowl and combine well.
2. Chill in the fridge before serving.

Nutrition: 118 calories per serving

Smoked salmon & chicory boats

Preparation time: 5 Minutes

Cooking Time: 25 Minutes

Servings: 4

Ingredients:

- 150g (5oz) red chicory leaves (or yellow if it's unavailable) 150g (5oz) smoked salmon, finely chopped 100g (3½oz) cucumber, diced
- 2 tablespoons fresh parsley, chopped ½ red onion, finely chopped
- Juice of 1 lime
- 2 tablespoons olive oil

Directions:

1. Place the salmon, cucumber, onion, parsley, oil and lime juice into a bowl and toss the ingredients well.
2. Scoop some of the salmon mixture into each of the chicory leaves and chill before serving.

Nutrition: 152 calories per serving

Vegetable Loaf

Preparation time: 5 Minutes

Cooking Time: 35 Minutes

Servings: 4

Ingredients:

- 175g (6oz) mushrooms, finely chopped 100g (3½ oz) haricot beans
- 100g (3½ oz) walnuts, finely chopped 100g (3½ oz) peanuts, finely chopped 1 carrot, finely chopped
- 3 sticks celery, finely chopped 1 bird's-eye chilli, finely chopped 1 red onion, finely chopped
- 1 egg, beaten
- 2 cloves of garlic, chopped
- 2 tablespoons olive oil
- 2 teaspoons turmeric powder
- 2 tablespoons soy sauce
- 4 tablespoons fresh parsley, chopped 100mls (3½ fl oz) water
- 60mls (2fl oz) red wine

Directions:

1. Heat the oil in a pan and add the garlic, chilli, carrot, celery, onion, mushrooms and turmeric.
2. Cook for 5 minutes.
3. Grease and line a large loaf tin with greaseproof paper.
4. Let it stand for 10 minutes then turn onto a serving plate.

Nutrition: 453 calories per serving

Dates ham

Preparation time: 5 Minutes

Cooking Time: 25 Minutes

Servings: 4

Ingredients:

1. 12 medjool dates
2. 2 slices of parma ham, cut into strips

Directions:

Wrap each date with a strip of parma ham.

Can be served hot or cold.

Nutrition: 202 calories per serving

Celery Breakfast

Preparation time: 5 Minutes

Cooking Time: 15 Minutes

Servings: 4

Ingredients:

- 250g (9oz) celery, chopped
- 100mls (3½ fl oz) warm vegetable stock (broth) 1 red onion, chopped
- 1 clove of garlic, crushed
- 1 tablespoon fresh parsley, chopped 25g (1oz) butter
- Sea salt and freshly ground black pepper

Directions:

1. Place the celery, onion, stock (broth) and garlic into a saucepan and simmer for 10 minutes.
2. Stir in the parsley and butter and season with salt and pepper.
3. Serve as an accompaniment to roast meat dishes

Nutrition: 67 calories

Cheesy Wheat cakes

Preparation time: 5 Minutes

Cooking Time: 30 Minutes

Servings: 4

Ingredients:

- 100g (3½oz) buckwheat, cooked and cooled 1 large egg

- 25g (1oz) cheddar cheese, grated (shredded) 25g (1oz) wholemeal breadcrumbs 2 shallots, chopped
- 2 tablespoons fresh parsley, chopped 1 tablespoon olive oil

Directions:

1. Crack the egg into a bowl, whisk it then set aside.
2. In a separate bowl, combine all the buckwheat, cheese, shallots, and parsley.
3. Mix well.
4. Pour in the beaten egg to the buckwheat mixture and stir well.
5. Shape the mixture into patties.
6. Scatter the breadcrumbs on a plate and roll the patties in them.
7. Heat the olive oil in a large frying pan.
8. And gently place the cakes in the oil.
9. Cook for 3-4 minutes on either side until slightly golden.

Nutrition: 358 calories

Red chicory cheese boats

Preparation time: 5 Minutes

Cooking Time: 25 Minutes

Servings: 4

Ingredients:

- 200g (7oz) stilton cheese, crumbled 200g (7oz) red chicory leaves (or if unavailable, use yellow) 2 tablespoon fresh parsley, chopped 1 tablespoon olive oil

Directions:

1. Place the red chicory leaves onto a baking sheet.

2. Drizzle them with olive oil then sprinkle the cheese inside the leaves.
3. Place them under a hot grill (broiler) for around 4 minutes.
4. Sprinkle with chopped parsley and serve straight away.

Nutrition: 250 calories

Turkey breakfast sausages

Preparation Time: 5 Minutes

Cooking time: 55 Minutes

Servings: 2

Ingredients:

- 1 lb extra lean ground turkey
- 1 tbsp EVOO 9 Extra Virgin Olive Oil) and a little more to coat pan
- 1 tbsp fennel seeds
- 2 teaspoons smoked paprika
- 1 teaspoon red pepper flakes
- 1 teaspoon peppermint
- 1 teaspoon chicken seasoning
- A couple of shredded cheddar cheese
- A couple of chives, finely chopped
- A few shakes garlic and onion powder
- Two spins of pepper and salt

Directions:

1. Preheat oven to 350 F.
2. Utilize a little EVOO to grease a miniature muffin pan.
3. Combine all ingredients and blend thoroughly.
4. Fill each pit on top of the pan and then cook for approximately 15-20 minutes.
5. Each toaster differs therefore when muffin temperature is 165 then remove.

Nutrition: 250 calories

Tuna, egg & caper salad

Preparation time: 5 Minutes

Cooking Time: 35 Minutes

Servings: 4

Ingredients:

- 100g (3½oz) red chicory (or yellow if not available) 150g (5oz) tinned tuna flakes in brine, drained 100g (3 ½ oz) cucumber
- 25g (1oz) rocket (arugula)
- 6 pitted black olives
- 2 hard-boiled eggs, peeled and quartered 2 tomatoes, chopped
- 2 tablespoons fresh parsley, chopped 1 red onion, chopped
- 1 stalk of celery
- 1 tablespoon capers
- 2 tablespoons garlic vinaigrette (see recipe)

Directions:

1. Place the tuna, cucumber, olives, tomatoes, onion, chicory, celery, parsley and rocket (arugula) into a bowl.
2. Pour in the vinaigrette and toss the salad in the dressing.
3. Serve onto plates and scatter the eggs and capers on top.

Nutrition: 340 calories

Hot chicory & nut salad

Preparation time: 5 Minutes

Cooking Time: 25 Minutes

Servings: 4

Ingredients:

For the salad:

- 100g (3½oz) green beans
- 100g (3½oz) red chicory, chopped (if unavailable use yellow chicory) 100g (3½oz) celery, chopped
- 25g (1oz) macadamia nuts, chopped 25g (1oz) walnuts, chopped
- 25g (1oz) plain peanuts, chopped 2 tomatoes, chopped
- 1 tablespoon olive oil
- For the dressing:
- 2 tablespoons fresh parsley, finely chopped ½ teaspoon turmeric
- ½ teaspoon mustard
- 1 tablespoon olive oil
- 25mls (1fl oz) red wine vinegar

Directions:

1. Mix together the ingredients for the dressing then set them aside.
2. Heat a tablespoon of olive oil in a frying pan then add the green beans, chicory and celery.
3. Cook until the vegetables have softened then add in the chopped tomatoes and cook for 2 minutes.
4. Add the prepared dressing and thoroughly coat all of the vegetables.
5. Serve onto plates and sprinkle the mixture of nuts over the top.
6. Eat immediately.

Nutrition: 438 calories

Honey chili squash

Preparation time: 5 Minutes

Cooking Time: 40 Minutes

Servings: 4

Ingredients:

- 2 red onions, roughly chopped 2.5cm (1 inch) chunk of ginger root, finely chopped 2 cloves of garlic
- 2 bird's-eye chillies, finely chopped 1 butternut squash, peeled and chopped 100mls (3½ fl oz) vegetable stock (broth) 1 tablespoon olive oil
- Juice of 1 orange
- Juice of 1 lime
- 2 teaspoons honey

Directions:

1. Warm the oil into a pan and add in the red onions, squash chunks, chillies, garlic, ginger and honey.
2. Cook for 3 minutes.
3. Squeeze in the lime and orange juice.
4. Pour in the stock (broth), orange and lime juice and cook for 15 minutes until tender.

Nutrition: 815 calories.

Lunch Recipes

King Prawn Stir-fry & Soba

Preparation Time: 15 minutes

Cooking Time: 20 mutes

Servings: 3-4 **servings**

Ingredients:

- 150g shelled raw king prawns, deveined
- 2 tsp. tamari
- 2 tsp. extra virgin olive oil
- 75 soba
- 1 garlic clove, finely chopped
- 1 bird's eye chili, finely chopped
- 1 tsp. finely chopped fresh ginger
- 20g red onions, sliced
- 40g celery, trimmed and sliced
- 75g green beans, chopped
- 50g kale, roughly chopped
- 100ml chicken stock

Directions:

1. Warm a skillet over a high heat.
2. Fry for the pawns in 1 tsp. Of the tamari and of olive oil.
3. Transfer the contents of the skillet to a plate.
4. Wipe the skillet with kitchen towel to remove the lingering sauce.
5. Boil water and cook the soba for 8 minutes.
6. Drain and set aside.
7. Using the remaining 1 tsp. Olive oil.
8. Fry the remaining ingredients for 3-4 minutes.
9. Make the stock boil, simmering until the vegetables are tender but still have bite.
10. Add the lovage, noodles and prawn into the skillet.
11. Stir, bring back to the boil and then serve.

Nutrition: 192 calories

Miso Caramelized Tofu

Preparation Time: 10 minutes

Cooking Time: 25

Servings: 3

Ingredients:

- 1 tbsp mirin
- 20g miso paste
- 1 * 150g firm tofu
- 40g celery, trimmed
- 35g red onion
- 120g courgette
- 1 bird's eye chili
- 1 garlic clove, finely chopped
- 1 tsp. finely chopped fresh ginger
- 50g kale, chopped
- 2 tsp. sesame seeds
- 35g buckwheat
- 1 tsp. ground turmeric
- 2 tsp. extra virgin olive oil
- 1 tsp. tamari or soy sauce

Directions:

1. Pre-heat your over to 200C or gas mark 6.

2. Cover a tray with baking parchment.
3. Combine the mirin and miso together.
4. Dice the tofu and coat it in the mirin-miso mixture in a resealable plastic bag.
5. Set aside to marinate.
6. Chop the vegetables.
7. Disperse the tofu across the lined tray and garnish with sesame seeds.
8. Roast for 20 minutes, or until caramelized.
9. Rinse the buckwheat using running water and a sieve.
10. Add to a pan of boiling water alongside turmeric.
11. Cook the buckwheat according to the packet instructions.
12. Heat the oil in a skillet over high heat.
13. Toss in the vegetables, herbs and spices then fry for 2-3 minutes.
14. Reduce to a medium heat and fry for a further 5 minutes.

Nutrition: 192 calories

Sirtfood Cauliflower Couscous & Turkey Steak

Preparation Time: 10 minutes

Cooking Time: 15 minutes

Servings: 2

Ingredients:

- 150g cauliflower, roughly chopped
- 1 garlic clove, finely chopped
- 40g red onion, finely chopped
- 1 bird's eye chili, finely chopped
- 1 tsp. finely chopped fresh ginger
- 2 tbsp extra virgin olive oil
- 2 tsp. ground turmeric
- 30g sun dried tomatoes, finely chopped
- 10g parsley

- 150g turkey steak
- 1 tsp. dried sage
- Juice of ½ lemon
- 1 tbsp capers

Directions:

1. Disintegrate the cauliflower using a food processor.
2. Blend in 1-2 pulses until the cauliflower has a breadcrumb-like consistency.
3. In a skillet, fry garlic, chili, ginger and red onion in 1 tsp. Olive oil.
4. Throw in the turmeric and cauliflower then cook for another 1-2 minutes.
5. Remove from heat and add the tomatoes and roughly half the parsley.
6. Garnish the turkey steak with sage and dress with oil.
7. In a skillet, over medium heat, fry the turkey steak for 5 minutes.
8. Once the steak is cooked add lemon juice, capers and a dash of water.
9. Stir and serve with the couscous.

Nutrition: 231 Calories

Mushroom & Tofu Scramble

Preparation Time: 10 minutes

Cooking Time: 10 minutes

Servings: 1

Ingredients:

- 100g tofu, extra firm
- 1 tsp. ground turmeric
- 1 tsp. mild curry powder
- 20g kale, roughly chopped
- 1 tsp. extra virgin olive oil
- 20g red onion, thinly sliced
- 50g mushrooms, thinly sliced
- 5g parsley, finely chopped

Directions:

1. Place 2 sheets of kitchen towel under and on-top of the tofu.
2. Then rest a considerable weight such as saucepan onto the tofu.
3. Ensure it drains off the liquid.
4. Combine the curry powder, turmeric and 1-2 tsp. of water.
5. Using a steamer cook kale for 3-4 minutes.
6. In a skillet, warm oil over a medium heat.
7. Add the chili, mushrooms and onion, cooking for several minutes.
8. Break the tofu into small pieces and toss in the skillet.
9. Coat with the spice paste and stir.
10. Cook for up to 5 minutes and fry for 2 more minutes.
11. Garnish with parsley before serving.

Nutrition: 232 calories

Prawn & Chili Pak Choi

Preparation Time: 10 minutes

Cooking Time: 10 minutes

Servings: 1

Ingredients:

- 75g brown rice
- 1 pak choi
- 60ml chicken stock
- 1 tbsp extra virgin olive oil
- 1 garlic clove, finely chopped
- 50g red onion, finely chopped
- ½ bird's eye chili, finely chopped
- 1 tsp. freshly grated ginger
- 125g shelled raw king prawns
- 1 tbsp soy sauce
- 1 tsp. five-spice
- 1 tbsp freshly chopped flat-leaf parsley
- A pinch of salt and pepper

Directions:

1. Bring a medium sized saucepan of water to the boil
2. and cook the brown rice for 25-30 minutes, or until softened.
3. Tear the pak choi into pieces.
4. Warm the chicken stock in a skillet over medium heat.
5. Toss in the pak choi, cooking until the pak choi has slightly wilted.
6. In another skillet, warm olive oil over high heat.
7. Toss in the ginger, chili, red onions and garlic frying for 2-3 minutes.
8. Throw in the pawns, five-spice and soy sauce.
9. Cook for 6-8 minutes, or until the cooked throughout.
10. Drain the brown rice and add to the skillet, stirring and cooking for 2-3 minutes.
11. Add the pak choi, garnish with parsley and serve.

Nutrition: 193 calories

Sirtfood Granola

Preparation Time: 10 minutes

Cooking Time: 25 minutes

Servings: 12

Ingredients:

- 200g oats
- 250g buckwheat flakes
- 100g walnuts, chopped
- 100g almonds, chopped
- 100g dried strawberries
- 1 ½ tsp. ground ginger

- 1 ½ tsp. ground cinnamon
- 120mls olive oil
- 2 tbsp honey

Directions:

1. Preheat your oven to 150C.
2. Line a tray with baking parchment.
3. Stir together walnuts, almonds, buckwheat flakes and oats with ginger and cinnamon.
4. In a large pan, warm olive oil and honey, heating until the honey has dissolved.
5. Pour the honey-oil over the other ingredients.
6. Stirring to ensuring an even coating.
7. Separate the granola evenly over the lined baking tray.
8. And roast for 50 minutes, or until golden.
9. Once cooled add the berries and store in an airtight container.
10. Eat dry or with milk and yogurt. It stays fresh for up to 1 week.

Nutrition: 231 calories

Tomato Frittata

Preparation Time: 10 minutes

Cooking Time: 15 minutes

Servings: 2

Ingredients:

- 50g cheddar cheese, grated
- 75g kalamata olives, pitted and halved
- 8 cherry tomatoes, halved
- 4 large eggs
- 1 tbsp fresh parsley, chopped
- 1 tbsp fresh basil, chopped
- 1 tbsp olive oil

Directions:

1. Whisk the eggs in a mixing bowl.
2. Toss in the parsley, basil, olives, tomatoes and cheese, stirring thoroughly.
3. Heat the olive oil over high heat.
4. Pour in the frittata mixture and cook for 5-10 minutes, or set.
5. Remove the skillet from the hob and place under the grill for 5 minutes, or until firm and set.
6. Divide into portions and serve immediately.

Nutrition: 231 calories

Horseradish Flaked Salmon Fillet & Kale

Preparation Time: 10 minutes

Cooking Time: 15 minutes

Servings: 2

Ingredients:

- 200g skinless, boneless salmon fillet
- 50g green beans
- 75g kale
- 1 tbsp extra virgin olive oil
- ½ garlic clove, crushed
- 50g red onion, chopped
- 1 tbsp fresh chives, chopped
- 1 tbsp freshly chopped flat-leaf parsley
- 1 tbsp low fat crème Fraiche
- 1tbsp horseradish sauce
- Juice of ¼ lemon
- A pinch of salt and pepper

Directions:

1. Preheat the grill.
2. Sprinkle a salmon fillet with salt and pepper.

3. Place under the grill for 10-15 minutes. Flake and set aside.
4. Using a steamer, cook the kale and green beans for 10 minutes.
5. In a skillet, warm the oil over a high heat.
6. Add garlic and red onion and fry for 2-3 minutes.
7. Toss in the kale and beans and then cook for 1-2 minutes more.
8. Mix the chives, parsley, crème fraiche, horseradish, lemon juice and flaked salmon.
9. Serve the kale and beans topped with the dressed flaked salmon.

Nutrition: 221 calories

Indulgent Yoghurt

Preparation Time: 10 minutes

Cooking Time: 15 minutes

Servings: 3

Ingredients:

- 125 mixed berries
- 150g Greek yoghurt
- 25 walnuts, chopped
- 10g dark chocolate at least 85% cocoa solids, grated

Directions:

1. Toss the mixed berries into a serving bowl.
2. Cover with yoghurt and top with chocolate and walnuts. Voila!

Nutrition: 231 calories

Tuna Salad

Preparation Time: 5 minutes

Cooking Time: 5 minutes

Servings: 1

Ingredients:

- 100g red chicory
- 150g tuna flakes in brine, drained
- 100g cucumber
- 25g rocket
- 6 kalamata olives, pitted
- 2 hard-boiled eggs, peeled and quartered
- 2 tomatoes, chopped
- 2 tbsp fresh parsley, chopped
- 1 red onion, chopped
- 1 celery stalk
- 1 tbsp capers
- 2 tbsp garlic vinaigrette

Directions:

1. Put the ingredients in a bowl and serve.

Nutrition: 245 calories

Chicken & Bean Casserole

Preparation Time: 10 minutes

Cooking Time: 15 minutes

Servings: 2

Ingredients:

- 400g 14oz chopped tomatoes
- 400g 14oz tinned cannellini beans or haricot beans
- 8 chicken thighs, skin removed
- 2 carrots, peeled and finely chopped
- 2 red onions, chopped
- 4 sticks of celery
- 4 large mushrooms
- 2 red peppers bell peppers, de-seeded and chopped

- 1 clove of garlic
- 2 tablespoons soy sauce
- 1 tablespoon olive oil
- liters 3 pints chicken stock broth

Directions:

1. Put and heat olive oil, add the garlic and onions and cook for 5 minutes.
2. Add in the chicken.
3. Cook for 5 minutes
4. Add the carrots, cannellini beans, celery, red peppers bell peppers and mushrooms.
5. Pour in the stock broth soy sauce and tomatoes.
6. Bring it to the boil, reduce the heat and simmer for 45 minutes.
7. Serve with rice or new potatoes.

Nutrition: 509 calories

Mussels in Red Wine Sauce

Preparation Time: 20 minutes

Cooking Time: 10 minutes

Servings: 2

Ingredients:

- 800g 2lb mussels
- 2 x 400g 14oz tins of chopped tomatoes
- 25g 1oz butter
- 1 tablespoon fresh chives, chopped
- 1 tablespoon fresh parsley, chopped
- 1 bird's-eye chili, finely chopped
- 4 cloves of garlic, crushed
- 400mls 14fl oz red wine
- Juice of 1 lemon

Directions:

1. Wash the mussels, remove their beards and set them aside.
2. Put butter in a saucepan. Add in the red wine.
3. Reduce the heat and add the parsley, chives, chili and garlic whilst stirring.
4. Add in the tomatoes, lemon juice and mussels.
5. Cover the saucepan and cook for 2-3.
6. Remove the saucepan from the heat.
7. Take out any mussels which haven't opened and discard them.
8. Serve and eat immediately.

Nutrition: 364 calories

Tuna and Kale

Preparation time: 5 minutes

Cooking time: 20 minutes

Servings: 4

Ingredients:

- 1 pound tuna fillets, boneless, skinless and cubed
- A pinch of salt and black pepper
- 2 tablespoons olive oil
- 1 cup kale, torn
- ½ cup cherry tomatoes, cubed
- 1 yellow onion, chopped

Directions:

1. Heat up a pan with the oil over medium heat.
2. Add the onion and sauté for 5 minutes.
3. Add the tuna and the other ingredients, toss.
4. Cook everything for 15 minutes more, divide between plates and serve.

Nutrition: calories 251, fat 4, fiber 7, carbs 14, protein 7

Lemongrass Mix

Preparation time: 10 minutes

Cooking time: 25 minutes

Servings: 4

Ingredients:

- 4 mackerel fillets, skinless and boneless
- 2 tablespoons olive oil
- 1 tablespoon ginger, grated
- 2 lemongrass sticks, chopped
- 2 red chilies, chopped
- Juice of 1 lime
- A handful parsley, chopped

Directions:

1. Combine the mackerel with the oil, ginger and the other ingredients.
2. Toss and bake at 390 degrees F for 25 minutes.
3. Divide everything between plates and serve.

Nutrition: calories 251, fat 3, fiber 4, carbs 14, protein 8

Scallops with Almonds and Mushrooms

Preparation time: 5 minutes

Cooking time: 10 minutes

Servings: 4

Ingredients:

- 1 pound scallops
- 2 tablespoons olive oil
- 4 scallions, chopped
- A pinch of salt and black pepper
- ½ cup mushrooms, sliced
- 2 tablespoon almonds, chopped
- 1 cup coconut cream

Directions:

1. Heat up a pan with the oil over medium heat, add the scallions and the mushrooms and sauté for 2 minutes.
2. Add the scallops and the other ingredients, toss, cook over medium heat for 8 minutes more, divide into bowls and serve.

Nutrition: calories 322, fat 23.7, fiber 2.2, carbs 8.1, protein 21.6

Scallops and Sweet Potatoes

Preparation time: 5 minutes

Cooking time: 22 minutes

Servings: 4

Ingredients:

- 1 pound scallops
- ½ teaspoon rosemary, dried
- ½ teaspoon oregano, dried
- 2 tablespoons avocado oil
- 1 yellow onion, chopped
- 2 sweet potatoes, peeled and cubed
- ½ cup chicken stock
- 1 tablespoon cilantro, chopped
- A pinch of salt and black pepper

Directions:

1. Heat up a pan with the oil over medium heat, add the onion and sauté for 2 minutes.
2. Add the sweet potatoes and the stock, toss and cook for 10 minutes more.
3. Add the scallops and the remaining ingredients, toss, cook for another 10 minutes, divide everything into bowls and serve.

Nutrition: calories 211, fat 2, fiber 4.1, carbs 26.9, protein 20.7

Salmon and Shrimp Salad

Preparation time: 5 minutes

Cooking time: 0 minutes

Servings: 4

Ingredients:

- 1 cup smoked salmon, boneless and flaked
- 1 cup shrimp, peeled, deveined and cooked
- ½ cup baby arugula
- 1 tablespoon lemon juice
- 2 spring onions, chopped
- 1 tablespoon olive oil
- A pinch of sea salt and black pepper

Directions:

1. In a salad bowl, combine the salmon with the shrimp and the other ingredients, toss and serve.

Nutrition: calories 210, fat 6, fiber 5, carbs 10, protein 12

Shrimp, Tomato and Dates Salad

Preparation time: 10 minutes

Cooking time: 0 minutes

Servings: 4

Ingredients:

- 1 pound shrimp, cooked, peeled and deveined
- 2 cups baby spinach
- 2 tablespoons walnuts, chopped
- 1 cup cherry tomatoes, halved
- 1 tablespoon lemon juice

- ½ cup dates, chopped
- 2 tablespoons avocado oil

Directions:

1. In a salad bowl, mix the shrimp with the spinach, walnuts and the other ingredients, toss and serve.

Nutrition: calories 243, fat 5.4, fiber 3.3, carbs 21.6, protein 28.3

Salmon and Watercress Salad

Preparation time: 10 minutes

Cooking time: 0 minutes

Servings: 4

Ingredients:

- 1 pound smoked salmon, boneless, skinless and flaked
- 2 spring onions, chopped
- 2 tablespoons avocado oil
- ½ cup baby arugula
- 1 cup watercress
- 1 tablespoon lemon juice
- 1 cucumber, sliced
- 1 avocado, peeled, pitted and roughly cubed
- A pinch of sea salt and black pepper

Directions:

1. In a salad bowl, mix the salmon with the spring onions, watercress and the other ingredients, toss and serve.

Nutrition: calories 261, fat 15.8, fiber 4.4, carbs 8.2, protein 22.7

Tuna and Tomatoes

Preparation time: 5 minutes

Cooking time: 20 minutes

Servings: 4

Ingredients:

- 1 yellow onion, chopped
- 1 tablespoon olive oil
- 1 pound tuna fillets, boneless, skinless and cubed
- 1 cup tomatoes, chopped
- 1 red pepper, chopped
- 1 teaspoon sweet paprika
- 1 tablespoon coriander, chopped

Directions:

1. Heat up a pan with the oil over medium heat
2. Add the onions and the pepper and cook for 5 minutes.
3. Add the other ingredients
4. Cook everything for 15 minutes.
5. Divide between plates and serve.

Nutrition: calories 215, fat 4, fiber 7, carbs 14, protein 7

Spinach and Kale Mix

Preparation time: 5 minutes

Servings: 4

Ingredients:

- 2 chopped shallots
- 1 c. no-salt-added and chopped canned tomatoes
- 2 c. baby spinach
- 2 minced garlic cloves
- 5 c. torn kale
- 1 tbsp. olive oil

Directions:

1. Heat up a pan with the oil over medium-high heat.

2. Add the shallots, stir and sauté for 5 minutes.
3. Add the spinach, kale and the other ingredients, toss.
4. Cook for 10 minutes more.
5. Divide between plates and serve.

Nutrition:

Calories: 89, Fat: 3.7 g, Carbs: 12.4 g, Protein: 3.6 g, Sugars: 0 g, Sodium: 50 mg

Turmeric Carrots

Preparation time: 10 minutes

Cooking time: 40 minutes

Servings: 4

Ingredients:

- 1 pound baby carrots, peeled
- 1 tablespoon olive oil
- 2 spring onions, chopped
- 2 tablespoons balsamic vinegar
- 2 garlic cloves, minced
- 1 teaspoon turmeric powder
- 1 tablespoon chives, chopped
- ¼ teaspoon cayenne pepper
- A pinch of salt and black pepper

Directions:

1. Spread the carrots on a baking sheet lined with parchment paper.
2. Add the oil, the spring onions and the other ingredients
3. Toss and bake at 380 degrees F for 40 minutes.
4. Divide the carrots between plates and serve.

Nutrition: calories 79, fat 3.8, fiber 3.7, carbs 10.9, protein 1

Spinach Mix

Preparation time: 10 minutes

Cooking time: 12 minutes

Servings: 4

Ingredients:

- 1 pound baby spinach
- 1 yellow onion, chopped
- 1 tablespoon olive oil
- 1 tablespoon lemon juice
- 2 garlic cloves, minced
- A pinch of cayenne pepper
- ¼ teaspoon smoked paprika
- A pinch of salt and black pepper

Directions:

1. Heat up a pan with the oil over medium-high heat
2. Add the onion and the garlic and sauté for 2 minutes.
3. Add the spinach and the other ingredients, toss.
4. Cook over medium heat for 10 minutes.
5. Divide between plates and serve as a side dish.

Nutrition: calories 71, fat 4, fiber 3.2, carbs 7.4, protein 3.7

Orange Carrots

Preparation time: 5 minutes

Cooking time: 25 minutes

Servings: 4

Ingredients:

- 1 pound carrots, peeled and roughly sliced
- 1 yellow onion, chopped
- 1 tablespoon olive oil
- Zest of 1 orange, grated
- Juice of 1 orange
- 1 orange, peeled and cut into segments
- 1 tablespoon rosemary, chopped
- A pinch of salt and black pepper

Directions:

1. Heat up a pan with the oil over medium-high heat
2. Add the onion and sauté for 5 minutes.
3. Add the carrots, the orange zest and the other ingredients, toss
4. Cook over medium heat for 20 minutes more
5. Divide between plates and serve.

Nutrition: calories 140, fat 3.9, fiber 5, carbs 26.1, protein 2.1

Greek Sea Bass Mix

Preparation time: 10 minutes

Cooking time: 22 minutes

Servings: 2

Ingredients:

- 2 sea bass fillets, boneless
- 1 garlic clove, minced
- 5 cherry tomatoes, halved
- 1 tablespoon chopped parsley
- 2 shallots, chopped
- Juice of ½ lemon
- 1 tablespoon olive oil
- 8 ounces baby spinach
- Cooking spray

Directions:

1. Grease a baking dish with cooking oil then add the fish, tomatoes, parsley and garlic.

2. Drizzle the lemon juice over the fish, cover the dish and place it in the oven at 350 degrees F.
3. Bake for 15 minutes and then divide between plates.
4. Heat up a pan with the olive oil over medium heat, add shallot, stir and cook for 1 minute.
5. Add spinach, stir, cook for 5 minutes more, add to the plate with the fish and serve.

Nutrition: calories 210, fat 3, fiber 6, carbs 10, protein 24

Creamy Asparagus Soup

Preparation time: 10 minutes

Cooking time: 0 minutes

Servings: 2

Ingredients:

- 8 ounces white mushrooms
- 12 asparagus spears, trimmed
- 1 avocado, pitted and peeled
- A pinch of salt and white pepper
- 1 yellow onion, peeled and chopped
- 3 cups water

Directions:

1. In your blender, add the mushrooms with asparagus, avocado, onion, water, salt and pepper.
2. Pulse well, divide into soup bowls and serve right away.
3. Heat if desired.
4. Enjoy!

Nutrition: calories 176, fat 3, fiber 9, carbs 16, protein 9

Mushroom Cream

Preparation time: 10 minutes

Cooking time: 0 minutes

Servings: 2

Ingredients:

- 2 tablespoons coconut aminos
- 1 tablespoon lime juice
- A pinch of sea salt and white pepper
- 1 cup white mushrooms
- 1 garlic clove, peeled
- 1 small yellow onion, chopped
- 2 cups cashew milk, unsweetened

Directions:

1. In your blender, mix mushrooms with garlic, onion, cashew milk, salt, pepper, lime juice and coconut aminos and pulse really well.
2. Divide into soup bowls and serve right away.
3. Enjoy!

Nutrition: calories 191, fat 2, fiber 6, carbs 14, protein 7

Tomato Cream

Preparation time: 10 minutes

Cooking time: 0 minutes

Servings: 2

Ingredients:

- 3 sun-dried tomato sliced
- 2 celery stalks, chopped
- 3 big tomatoes, chopped
- ½ teaspoon powdered onion
- 2 basil springs, chopped
- ½ teaspoon garlic powder
- 1 small avocado, pitted and peeled

- A pinch of sea salt and white pepper

Directions:

1. In your blender, add the tomatoes with celery, onion powder, garlic powder, basil, avocado, salt and pepper and pulse really well.
2. Add sun-dried tomatoes and blend again until smooth.
3. Divide into soup bowls and serve.
4. Enjoy!

Nutrition: calories 167, fat 11, fiber 9, carbs 14, protein 4

Zucchini Pan

Preparation time: 5 minutes

Cooking time: 20 minutes

Servings: 4

Ingredients:

1. 1 pound zucchinis, sliced
2. 1 yellow onion, chopped
3. 2 tablespoons olive oil
4. 2 apples, peeled, cored and cubed
5. 1 tomato, cubed
6. 1 tablespoon rosemary, chopped
7. 1 tablespoon chives, chopped

Directions:

1. Heat up a pan with the oil over medium heat
2. Add the onion and sauté for 5 minutes.
3. Add the zucchinis and the other ingredients, toss.
4. Cook over medium heat for 15 minutes more.
5. Divide between plates and serve as a side dish.

Nutrition: calories 170, fat 5, fiber 2, carbs 11, protein 7

Ginger Mushrooms

Preparation time: 10 minutes

Cooking time: 20 minutes

Servings: 4

Ingredients:

- 1 pound mushrooms, sliced
- 1 yellow onion, chopped
- 1 tablespoon ginger, grated
- 1 tablespoon olive oil
- 2 tablespoons balsamic vinegar
- 2 garlic cloves, minced
- A pinch of salt and black pepper
- ¼ cup lime juice
- 2 tablespoons walnuts, chopped

Directions:

1. Heat up a pan with the oil over medium-high heat.
2. Add the onion and the ginger and sauté for 5 minutes.
3. Add the mushrooms and the other ingredients, toss.
4. Cook over medium heat for 15 minutes more.
5. Divide between plates and serve.

Nutrition: calories 120, fat 2, fiber 2, carbs 4, protein 5

Salmon fillet, endive, arugula and celery

Preparation time: 10 minutes

Cooking time: 20 minutes

Servings: 4

Ingredients:

- 200g fresh salmon fillet
- 200g arugula
- Three red endives
- One large pink grapefruit
- Two slices of smoked salmon
- One small shallot
- One lemon
- Grated Parmesan cheese
- Extra virgin olive oil
- One teaspoon balsamic vinegar
- Salt and pepper to taste

Directions:

1. Cut the lemon in half to gently extract the liquid juice inside it.
2. Peel the grapefruit over a bowl to collect the juice.
3. Detach the quarters and cut them into pieces.
4. Peel and chop the shallot.
5. Remove the skin and bones from the fresh salmon fillet, then dice into small pieces
6. Place the whole mixture in a salad bowl, sprinkle with the lime and grapefruit juice, mix and let stand aside.
7. Cut the bottoms of the endives, remove the damaged leaves and chop the main parts into thin strips.
8. Wash and wring the arugula.
9. Carefully cut the smoked salmon slices into light strips.
10. Drain the marinated salmon fillet well and keep two teaspoons of the marinade.
11. Emulsify the marinade with olive oil and balsamic vinegar in a bowl, then salt and pepper as desired.
12. In a salad bowl, mix the diced salmon fillet, the smoked salmon strips, the pieces of grapefruit, the arugula, the minced endives and the olive oil sauce
13. Turn to mix and sprinkle lightly with grated Parmesan cheese.
14. Serve this salad immediately and serve with slices of toast.
15. Do not hesitate to double the proportions if you want to enjoy it as a main dish.

Nutrition: calories 120, fat 2, fiber 2, carbs 4 protein 5

Tuscan bean stew

Preparation time: 10 minutes

Cooking time: 20 minutes

Servings: 4

Ingredients:

- Two teaspoons extra virgin olive oil
- 6 oz. cooked chicken sausages cut lengthwise in half and sliced
- 10 oz. fresh mushrooms
- One small raw red onion
- Two thinly sliced garlic cloves
- 29 oz. canned, diced tomatoes
- Sixteen oz. canned beans
- One medium uncooked zucchini
- One tbsp. rosemary
- ¼ tsp salt
- 2 oz. arugula
- ¼ cups Grated Parmesan Cheese

Directions:

1. By using a Dutch oven, set the heat level to medium-high.
2. Add the sausages and cook, often stirring, until lightly browned, about three minutes.
3. Using a cooking spoon, transfer to a small bowl or plate.

4. Add the mushrooms and onion to the pot and cook, often stirring, until the vegetables are tender, usually for about three minutes.
5. Now add the garlic and cook, constantly stirring for about 30 seconds.
6. Add the sausages to the tomatoes, beans, zucchini, rosemary and salt and allow to boil.
7. Lower the heat and simmer, till the mushrooms becomes soft, usually after about 2 minutes.
8. Remove from heat and stir in the arugula until it is softened.
9. Pour the stew into four bowls and garnish evenly with Parmesan.

Nutrition: calories 120, fat 2, fiber 2, carbs 4, protein 5

Strawberry buckwheat salad

Preparation time: 10 minutes

Cooking time: 20 minutes

Servings: 4

Ingredients:

Tamari dressing:

- One-quarter cup of olive oil
- Two tablespoons of vinegar
- One tablespoon of reduced salt tamari sauce
- One tablespoon of old-fashioned mustard
- Salad:
- One cup buckwheat, rinsed and drained
- 6 cups mixed lettuce
- 2 cups strawberries, hulled and sliced
- A half fennel bulb cut into thin slices
- One-third cup of red onion, cut into thin strips
- Six cooked bacon slices, chopped

- One-third cup of roasted sunflower seeds
- Salt and pepper

Directions:

Tamari vinaigrette

1. In a small jar, put the olive oil, rice vinegar, tamari sauce and old-fashioned mustard.
2. Add in some pepper.
3. Close the lid and shake vigorously.
4. Salad preparation
5. Now place the buckwheat in a medium-sized bowl and cover with at least 2 inches (5 cm) of water.
6. Cover the bowl and let soak in the refrigerator overnight.
7. Drain buckwheat, rinse with cold water and drain again.
8. In a large bowl, put the lettuce, strawberries, fennel, onion, bacon, sunflower seeds and reserved buckwheat.
9. Add in your dressing and mix well.

Nutrition: calories 120, fat 2, fiber 2, carbs 4, protein 5

Sautéed potatoes in chicken broth

Preparation time: 10 minutes

Cooking time: 20 minutes

Servings: 4

Ingredients:

- Six medium-sized potatoes
- One onion
- Chicken broth
- 100ml of water
- One tbsp extra virgin olive oil
- Salt to taste

Directions:

1. First peel the potatoes then slice it across into pieces.
2. Proceed by peeling the onions and chop into small pieces.
3. Fry minced onion pieces in oil for five minutes.
4. Add in the potatoes and cook for another ten minutes while stirring gently.
5. Dilute the chicken broth with water and add to the cooker and cook for five minutes.
6. Add salt to taste and serve.

Nutrition: calories 120, fat 2, fiber 2, carbs 4,

protein 5

Baked potatoes and chili con carne

Preparation time: 10 minutes

Cooking time: 20 minutes

Servings: 4

Ingredients:

- 8Big potatoes
- 600g Knife ground beef
- 35cl Beef broth
- 500g Crushed tomatoes
- 500g Canned kidney beans
- 1 tbsp. Tomato puree
- 2 Big onions
- One bunch of chives
- Two garlic cloves
- Half teaspoon Chili powder
- One tbsp. Cumin
- One tbsp. dried oregano
- 2 tbsp. Extra Virgin Olive Oil
- 250g Farm fresh cream
- Salt and pepper to taste

Directions:

1. Peel and chop the onions and garlic.
2. Heat the broth in a saucepan.
3. Heat the oil available in the frying pan to fry the onions and garlic for five minutes while mixing.
4. Add the meat and allow to cook for five minutes over high heat.
5. Add salt and pepper.
6. Pour the tomatoes and the tomato puree, then the broth.
7. Add the cumin, oregano and chili and then mix.
8. Cover and simmer 45 minutes.
9. Add the beans, cover and continue cooking over low heat, 20 min.
10. Preheat the oven to 180 ° C
11. Wash the potatoes. Once done, wrap them together in aluminum foil and bake for 30 to 35 minutes.
12. Remove the paper, cut the potatoes in half and scoop it out slightly to garnish with chili.
13. Top each potato with a spoonful of cream
14. Serve hot.

Nutrition: calories 120, fat 2, fiber 2, carbs 4, protein 5

Chicken in pepper sauce

Preparation time: 10 minutes

Cooking time: 20 minutes

Servings: 4

Ingredients:

- One jar of 340 ml roasted peppers
- One cup (250 mL) canned coconut milk
- Fifteen ml red wine vinegar
- Two cloves of garlic
- One tsp. paprika

- One tsp. dried oregano
- One tsp. salt
- One-quarter cup of chopped fresh parsley, chopped
- One tbsp extra virgin olive oil
- Four boneless skinless chicken breasts or thighs
- Salt and pepper
- One minced onion
- One red bell pepper (minced)
- One-quarter cup of chopped fresh parsley, for garnish

Directions:

1. In a blender, mix all the ingredients for the sauce (everything above except chicken, olive oil, onions, salt and pepper) until you get a mixture of smooth consistency.
2. Place a rack at the center of your oven and preheat to 400 ° F.
3. In your large non-stick skillet (you can use a cast iron), heat the olive oil over high heat and fry the chicken breasts.
4. Generously season with salt and pepper.
5. Give it time by allowing all the sides of the chicken to fry for at least three minutes and then set aside on a plate.
6. Lower the heat level back to medium then add the onions and allow to heat for six minutes over medium heat, stirring often.
7. Add the red pepper and cook for another minute only.
8. Return the chicken to the pan and sprinkle with the roasted pepper sauce.
9. Bake the dish for fifteen minutes.
10. Before serving, remove from the oven and grace it by adding some parsley.
11. Serve with pasta in olive oil and chives or white rice.

Nutrition: calories 120, fat 2, fiber 2, carbs 4, protein 5

Waldorf salad

Preparation time: 10 minutes

Cooking time: 20 minutes

Servings: 4

Ingredients:

- One hundred and twenty-five grams of mayonnaise
- Two tablespoons white vinegar
- One apple, peeled and cut into pieces
- One celery stalk, diced
- One hundred and twenty-five grams of grapes
- One hundred and twenty-five grams of chopped walnuts
- Salt and pepper to taste

Directions:

1. In a large bowl, whisk the mayonnaise and vinegar.
2. Add the apple, celery, raisins and walnuts.
3. Sprinkle in salt and pepper. Mix everything and serve fresh.

Nutrition: calories 120, fat 2, fiber 2, carbs 4, protein 5

Whole wheat pita

Preparation time: 10 minutes

Cooking time: 20 minutes

Servings: 4

Ingredients:

- 250g of whole wheat flour
- 2 tbsp extra virgin olive oil

- 5g salt
- 10g dry baker's yeast
- One hundred and fifty-ml hot water

Directions:

1. Add the whole flour and the salt in a bowl and stir.
2. Then add the rest of the ingredients: oil, yeast and water.
3. Stir thoroughly to mix.
4. Mix all the ingredients well until the pita bread dough is formed.
5. Knead the dough for a few minutes on the table.
6. If the dough seems to be too dry, you can add a little more water.
7. Once kneaded, make the dough into a ball and put it in a bowl.
8. Have it covered and let it be there for two hours.
9. Take out the whole pita bread dough and knead again.
10. Work the dough into balls of about 80g each.
11. Use a roller to make the dough well-rounded.
12. Make the pieces of bread ten-to-twelve cm wide and One cm thick.
13. Put the pitas on a tray.
14. Preheat the oven to 200 ° C, slot in the tray and let the pieces of bread bake for ten minutes, depending on the oven.
15. Finally, take out the pieces of bread, let them cool a little and serve!

Nutrition: calories 120, fat 2, fiber 2, carbs 4, protein 5

Scrambled tofu with mushrooms (vegan)

Preparation time: 10 minutes

Cooking time: 20 minutes

Servings: 4

Ingredients:

- One hundred and twenty-five grams of plain firm tofu
- 100g silky tofu
- One tbsp. fresh cream
- One tbsp. sesame puree
- One tsp. Mustard
- ½ tsp. ground turmeric
- Four sprigs of fresh chives
- Half onion (optional)
- One garlic clove (optional)
- 50g mushrooms
- 2 tbsp. Extra Virgin Olive Oil
- One tbsp. Tamari soy sauce (gluten-free, organic soy sauce)
- Salt and pepper to taste

Directions:

1. In a bowl, crush the firm tofu, add in the silky tofu, cream, tahini, mustard, turmeric and chopped chives.
2. Mix thoroughly and add salt and pepper to taste.
3. Peel and chop the onion and the garlic.
4. Rinse the mushrooms under a stream of water.
5. Cut off the ends of the stalks and cut the mushrooms into strips.
6. Gently fry the mushrooms, onionsand garlic over medium-high heat in a pan with a little olive oil.
7. Once the mushrooms, onionsand garlic are very tender and slightly brown in color, add the mixture to the tofu and cook over medium heat for about 5 minutes.
8. Stir the mixture continuously with a spatula.
9. Serve hotand enjoy.

Nutrition: calories 120, fat 2, fiber 2, carbs 4, protein 5

Pasta with smoked salmon and arugula

Preparation time: 10 minutes

Cooking time: 20 minutes

Servings: 4

Ingredients:

- 250g Spaghetti
- One hundred and fifty grams of Smoked salmon
- One bunch of arugula
- 2 tbsp. Extra virgin olive oil
- One finely chopped onion
- Salt and pepper to taste

Directions:

1. Cook the pasta in boiling water for ten minutes.
2. Add salt to taste.
3. Slice the smoked salmon into strips.
4. Rinse and wring the arugula.
5. Heat One tablespoonful of extra virgin olive oil in a frying pan and chop the onion.
6. Add in the drained spaghetti, the salmon strips and the arugula.
7. Mix well and cook for 2 min.
8. Sprinkle in the rest of the olive oil, salt and pepper.
9. Mix and serve hot.

Nutrition: calories 120, fat 2, fiber 2, carbs 4, protein 5

Sirtfood Chicken Breasts

Preparation time: 10 minutes

Cooking time: 20 minutes

Servings: 4

Ingredients:

- Chicken breasts, 5 oz
- Chopped Kale, 1 cup
- Red Onion, sliced, ½ cup
- Buckwheat, 1 cup
- Fresh ginger, chopped, 1 tsp
- Olive Oil, extra virgin, 1 tbsp
- Turmeric, ground, 2 tsp
- ¼ lemon, juiced
- Salsa
- Tomato, chopped, 1 cup
- 1 chopped bird's eye's chili
- Capers, finely chopped, 1 tbsp
- Parsley, finely chopped, 1 tsp
- ¼ lemon, juiced

Directions:

1. Chop the tomato while making sure not to squish it and preserve the maximum liquid in the process.
2. Add the lemon juice, parsley, capers and chili.
3. Pop everything into a blender and you're done!
4. Heat your oven to 220 °C.
5. While your oven is heating, marinate the chicken with turmeric, olive oil and the lemon juice up to 15 minutes.
6. Cook in an ovenproof pan on each side until the chicken turns pale golden.
7. Transfer to the oven and bake for 10 minutes, cover with foil and cook for another five minutes.
8. While your chicken is baking, steam the kale for five minutes, adding red onions, ginger and little oil.
9. Mix and fry for up to five minutes.
10. To make the second side dish, cook buckwheat with turmeric according to

instructions on the package and serve all together.

Nutrition: calories 120, fat 2, fiber 2, carbs 4, protein 5

Turkey With Sirtfood Vegetables

This recipe is highly adjustable and it's based on combining turkey as the main dish with healthy side-dishes made of vegetables. It's extremely simple and convenient, as meats go great with any and all Sirt spices and vegetables. With that in mind, feel free to adjust or replace any ingredient in this recipe with an equal amount of the ingredients you prefer or like better.

Preparation time: 10 minutes

Cooking time: 20 minutes

Servings: 4

Ingredients:

- Lean turkey meat, 150 g
- 1 finely chopped garlic clove
- 1 finely chopped red onion
- 1 finely chopped bird's eye chili/replace with chopped red bell paprika or ½ squeezed citrus fruit if you don't like spicy foods
- 1 tsp of finely chopped ginger
- Extra virgin olive oil, 2 tbsp
- Ground turmeric, 1 tbsp
- ½ cup of dried tomatoes
- Parsley, 10 g
- Sage, dried, 1 tsp
- ½ juiced lime or lemon
- Capers, 1 tbsp

Directions:

1. Chop the cauliflower.
2. Fry with chopped ginger, chili, red onion and garlic in 1 tbsp olive oil until they're soft.
3. Add cauliflower and turmeric and cook for a couple of minutes until the cauliflower becomes soft.
4. Once the dish is done, add dried tomatoes and parsley.
5. Coat your turkey in a thin layer of olive oil and sage.
6. Fry for about five minutes and then add the capers and lime juice to the mix.
7. Add half a cup of water and bring to a boil.

Nutrition: calories 120, fat 2, fiber 2, carbs 4, protein 5

Sirtfood Beans With Beef

Preparation time: 10 minutes

Cooking time: 20 minutes

Servings: 4

Ingredients:

- Kidney beans, 2 small cans
- Lean beef, minced, 400 g
- Buckwheat, 160 g
- 1 finely chopped red onion
- 1 chopped red bell pepper
- Two finely chopped bird's eye chili peppers
- Canned tomatoes, 800 g
- Ground turmeric, 1 tbsp
- Tomato sauce, 1 tbsp
- Cocoa powder, 1 tbsp
- Ground cumin, 1 tbsp
- Extra virgin olive oil, 1 tbsp
- Red wine, 150 ml
- Chopped coriander, ½ tbsp.
- Chopped parsley, ½ tbsp.

Directions:

1. Fry the onions, chili peppers and garlic for three minutes over medium heat.
2. Throw in the spices and mince for another minute.
3. After that, add the beef and red wine.
4. Bring to a boil and let it bubble until the liquid reduces by a half.
5. Add the cocoa powder, tomatoes, tomato sauce and the red bell pepper.
6. Add more water if needed and let the dish simmer on low medium heat for an hour.
7. Add the remaining chopped herbs before serving.

Nutrition: calories 120, fat 2, fiber 2, carbs 4, protein 5

Chicken and Kale Buckwheat Noodles

This tasty dish will take no more than 30 minutes to prepare, prep time included.

Preparation time: 10 minutes

Cooking time: 20 minutes

Servings: 4

Ingredients:

For noodles

- Finely chopped kale, 2 cups
- Buckwheat noodles, 5 oz
- Shiitake mushrooms (or any other of your choosing), four pieces
- Extra virgin olive oil, 1 tsp
- 1 finely diced red onion
- 1 diced chicken breast
- 1 sliced bird's eye chili
- Soy sauce, 3 tbsp

Salad dressing

- Soy sauce, ¼ cup
- Tamari sauce, 1 tbsp
- Sesame oil, 1 tbsp
- Lemon juice, 1 tbsp

Directions:

1. Boil or stir-fry chicken for up to 15 minutes.
2. Microwave kale up to three minutes to preserve nutrients.
3. Cook buckwheat noodles and rinse and add kale once they're done.
4. Fry the mushrooms with 1 tsp of olive oil up to three minutes and season with a pinch of salt.
5. Set aside and use the same pan, adding more olive oil, to sauté peppers and chickpeas up to five minutes.
6. Add garlic, water and tamari sauce and cook for another three minutes.
7. Add kale with noodles, chickenand dressing.
8. Mix all together and serve.

Nutrition: calories 120, fat 2, fiber 2, carbs 4, protein 5

Sirtfood Lamb

Preparation time: 10 minutes

Cooking time: 20 minutes

Servings: 4

Ingredients:

- Extra virgin olive oil, 2 tbsp
- Grated ginger, one inch
- 1 sliced red onion.
- 1 tsp of bird's eye
- Cumin seeds, 2 tsp
- 1 cinnamon stick
- Lamb, 800 g
- Garlic cloves, crushed, 3 pieces

- A pinch of salt
- Chopped Medjool dates, 1 cup
- Chickpeas, 400 g
- Coriander, 2 tbsp
- Buckwheat

Directions:

1. Start by preheating your oven to 140 °C.
2. Sauté sliced onion with 2 tbsp of extra virgin olive oil for five minutes while keeping the lid on.
3. The onions should turn soft but not brown.
4. Add turmeric, cumin, ginger, garlic and chili and stir fry for another minute.
5. Add the chunks of lamb, season with salt and letand let boil.
6. Add a glass of water.
7. After the mixture has boiled, roast in the oven for one hour and 15 minutes.
8. Add the chickpeas half an hour before the dish is finished.
9. Add chopped coriander and serve with buckwheat after the meal is done.

Nutrition: calories 120, fat 2, fiber 2, carbs 4, protein 5

Fish With Mango and Turmeric

Preparation time: 10 minutes

Cooking time: 20 minutes

Servings: 4

Ingredients:

- A fresh 1 ¼ lbs piece of fish of your choosing
- ½ cup of coconut oil
- A pinch of sea salt
- 1 tbsp of high-quality red wine
- ¼ cup olive oil
- ½ tbsp minced ginger

- Scallion, 2 cups
- Dill, 2 cups
- 1 ripe mango
- 1 squeezed lemon
- 1 garlic clove
- Dry red pepper, 1 tsp
- Fresh cilantro
- Walnuts

Directions:

1. Marinate the fish and leave overnight
2. Blend the ingredients for mango dipping sauce
3. Fry the fish in 2 tbsp in coconut oil on medium heat and add a pinch of salt after five minutes.
4. Turn to the other side and fry for another couple of minutes.
5. Keep the remaining oil in the pan.
6. Add scallions and dill and turn off the heat.
7. Heat for about 15 seconds and season with a pinch of salt.
8. Top the fish with the infused oil, dilland scallion and serve with the mango sauce, nuts, limeand cilantro.

Nutrition: calories 120, fat 2, fiber 2, carbs 4, protein 5

Sirtfood Shrimp Noodles

Preparation time: 10 minutes

Cooking time: 20 minutes

Servings: 4

Ingredients:

- Shrimps, deveined 1/3 lb.
- Soy sauce, 2 tsp
- Extra virgin olive oil, 2 tsp
- Buckwheat noodles, 3oz
- 2 finely chopped garlic cloves

- 1 bird's eye chili, finely chopped
- Chopped fresh ginger, 1 tsp
- Chopped red onion, ¼
- Chopped celery with eaves, ½ cup
- Chopped green beans, ½ cup
- Chopped kale, 1 cup
- Chicken stock, ½ cup

Directions:

1. Cook the shrimps in 1 tsp of the soy sauce and one tsp of the oil up to three minutes on high heat.
2. Cook buckwheat noodles for up to eight minutes and drain.
3. Fry the remaining ingredients in a pan on medium heat for up to three minutes.
4. Add the chicken stock, bring to a boiland cook until the veggies are cooked, but still look fresh.
5. Add the shrimps and noodles, bring to a boiland you're done!

Nutrition: calories 120, fat 2, fiber 2, carbs 4, protein 5

Sirtfood Miso Salmon

Preparation time: 10 minutes

Cooking time: 20 minutes

Servings: 4

Ingredients:

- Miso, ½ cup
- Organic red wine, 1 tbsp
- Extra virgin olive oil, 1 tbsp
- Salmon, 7 oz
- 1 sliced red onion
- Celery, sliced, 1 cup
- 2 finely chopped garlic cloves
- 1 finely chopped bird's eye chili
- Ground turmeric, 1 tsp
- Freshly chopped ginger, 1 tsp

- Green beans, 1 cup
- Kale, finely chopped, 1 cup
- Sesame seeds. 1 tsp
- Soy sauce, 1 tbsp
- Buckwheat, 2 tbsp

Directions:

1. Marinate the salmon in the mix of red wine, 1 tsp of extra virgin olive oiland miso for 30 minutes.
2. Preheat your oven to 420 °F and bake the fish for ten minutes.
3. Fry the onions, chili, garlic, green beans, ginger, kaleand celery for a few minutes until it's cooked.
4. Insert the soy sauce, parsley and sesame seeds.
5. Cook buckwheat per instructions and mix in with the stir-fry.
6. Enjoy!

Nutrition: calories 120, fat 2, fiber 2, carbs 4, protein 5

Sirtfood Shrimps With Buckwheat Noodles

Preparation time: 10 minutes

Cooking time: 20 minutes

Servings: 4

Ingredients:

- Shrimps (or a piece of fish of your choosing), 4 oz
- Tamari, 2 tbsp
- Extra virgin olive oil, 2 tbsp
- Buckwheat noodles, 75 g
- 1 finely chopped bird's eye chili
- 1 finely chopped garlic clove
- Fresh ginger, chopped, 1 tsp
- 1 sliced red onion
- Sliced red celery, ½ cup

- Chopped green beans, 1 cup
- Chopped kale, 1 cup
- Chicken stock, 1 cup
- Celery, 1 tsp

Directions:

1. Cook the shrimps for three minutes on high heat and with 1 tsp of tamari and 1 tsp of extra virgin olive oil.
2. Set aside.
3. Cook the noodles for up to eight minutes and set aside.
4. Fry kale, beans, celeryand onion, ginger, chiliand garlic in oil for up to three minutes.
5. Add vegetable stock and simmer for two minutes.
6. Mix all together, bring to a boiland serve.

Sirtfood Shellfish Salad

Preparation time: 10 minutes

Cooking time: 20 minutes

Servings: 4

Ingredients:

- Tomato sauce, 1 tsp
- Cloves, ¼ tsp
- Coriander, chopped, 1 tbsp
- Parsley, chopped, 1 tbsp
- Lemon juice, 1 tbsp (½ of a lemon)
- Kale, chopped, 1 cup
- Spinach, chopped, 1 cup
- Sea fruit of your choosing (shrimps, prawns, or clamps), 1 cup
- Chopped firm tofu, 1 thick slice (approx. 4 oz)
- Buckwheat noodles, 1 cup
- Pecan nuts, ½ cup
- Chopped ginger, ½ cup

- Miso paste, 1 tbsp
- Carrots, ½ cup
- Chicken stock, 100 ml

Directions:

1. Simmer tomato sauce with lemon juice, chicken stock, coriander, parsley and shrimps/cloves/clams for 10 minutes on medium heat.
2. Add the remaining ingredients without the ginger and miso and stir-fry until the shellfish is cooked through.
3. Add the remaining seasonings and you're done!

Nutrition: calories 120, fat 2, fiber 2, carbs 4, protein 5

Coq Au Vin

Preparation time: 15 minutes

Cooking time: 1 hour 15 minutes

Servings: 8

Ingredients:

- 450g button mushrooms
- 100g streaky bacon, chopped
- 16 chicken thighs, skin removed
- 3 cloves of garlic, crushed
- 3g fresh parsley, chopped
- 3 carrots, chopped
- 2 red onions, chopped
- 2 tablespoons plain flour
- 2 teaspoons olive oil
- 750mls red wine
- 1 bouquet garnish

Directions:

1. Place the flour on a large plate and coat the chicken in it.

2. Heat the olive oil in a large saucepan, add the chicken and brown it, before setting aside.
3. Fry the bacon in the pan then add the onion and cook for 5 minutes.
4. Pour in the red wine and add the chicken, carrots, bouquet garnish and garlic.
5. Transfer it to a large ovenproof dish.
6. Cook in the oven at 180C/360F for 1 hour.
7. Remove the bouquet garnish and skim off any excess fat, if necessary.
8. Add in the mushrooms and cook for 15 minutes.
9. Stir in the parsley just before serving.

Nutrition:

Calories: 459

Net carbs: 66g

Fat: 1g

Fiber: 4g8g

Protein:

Moroccan Chicken Casserole

Preparation time: 20 minutes

Cooking time: 50 minutes

Servings: 4

Ingredients:

- 4 chicken breasts, cubed
- 250g tinned chickpeas (garbanzo beans) drained
- 4 medjool dates, halved
- 6 dried apricots, halved
- 1 red onion, sliced 1 carrot, chopped
- 1 teaspoon ground cumin
- 1 teaspoon ground cinnamon
- 1 teaspoon ground turmeric

- 1 bird's-eye chili, chopped
- 600mls chicken stock
- 25g corn flour 60mls water
- 2 teaspoons fresh coriander

Directions:

1. Place the chicken, chickpeas (garbanzo beans), onion, carrot, chili, cumin, turmeric, cinnamon and stock (broth) into a large saucepan.
2. In a cup, mix the corn flour together with the water until it becomes a smooth paste.
3. Pour the mixture into the saucepan and stir until it thickens.
4. Add in the coriander (cilantro) and mix well.
5. Serve with buckwheat or couscous.

Nutrition: Calories: 401 Net carbs: 3.6g

Fat: 4.8g Fiber: 1.7g Protein: 29.2g

Prawn and Coconut Curry

Preparation time: 10 minutes

Cooking time: 5 minutes

Servings: 4

Ingredients:

- 400g tinned chopped tomatoes
- 400g large prawns (shrimps), shelled and raw
- 25g fresh coriander (cilantro) chopped
- 3 red onions, finely chopped
- 3 cloves of garlic, crushed
- 2 bird's eye chilies
- ½ teaspoon ground coriander (cilantro)
- ½ teaspoon turmeric
- 400mls (14fl Oz) coconut milk
- 1 teaspoons olive oil
- Juice of 1 lime

Directions:

1. Place the onions, garlic, tomatoes, chilies, lime juice, turmeric, ground coriander (cilantro), chilies and half of the fresh coriander (cilantro) into a blender and blitz until you have a smooth curry paste.
2. Heat the olive oil in a frying pan, add the paste and cook for 2 minutes.
3. Stir in the coconut milk and warm it thoroughly.
4. Add the prawns (shrimps) to the paste and cook them until they have turned pink and are completely cooked.
5. Stir in the fresh coriander (cilantro).
6. Serve with rice.

Nutrition: Calories: 322 Net carbs: 98.9g

Fat: 11.8g Fiber: 8g Protein: 15.6g

Chicken and Bean Casserole

Preparation time: 15 minutes

Cooking time: 55 minutes

Servings: 4

Ingredients:

- 400g chopped tomatoes
- 400g tinned cannellini beans or haricot beans
- 8 chicken thighs, skin removed
- 2 carrots, peeled and finely chopped
- 2 red onions, chopped
- 4 sticks of celery
- 4 large mushrooms
- 2 red peppers (bell peppers), de-seeded and chopped
- 1 clove of garlic
- 2 teaspoons soy sauce
- 1 olive oil
- liters chicken stock (broth)

Directions:

1. Heat the olive oil in a saucepan.
2. Add the garlic and onions and cook for 5 minutes.
3. Add in the chicken.
4. And cook for 5 minutes.
5. Add the carrots, cannellini beans, celery, red peppers (bell peppers) and mushrooms.
6. Pour in the stock (broth) soy sauce and tomatoes.
7. Bring it to the boil, reduce the heat and simmer for 45 minutes.
8. Serve with rice or new potatoes.

Nutrition: Calories: 509 Net carbs: 12.5g

Fat: 6.5g Fiber: 1.1g Protein: 27.4g

Mussels in Red Wine Sauce

Preparation time: 5 minutes

Cooking time: 5 minutes

Servings: 2

Ingredients:

- 800g mussels
- 2 x 400g tins of chopped tomatoes
- 25g butter
- 1 fresh chives, chopped
- 1 fresh parsley, chopped
- 1 bird's-eye chili, finely chopped
- 4 cloves of garlic, crushed
- 400mls red wine
- Juice of 1 lemon

Directions:

1. Wash the mussels, remove their beards and set them aside.
2. Heat the butter in a large saucepan and add in the red wine.

3. Reduce the heat and add the parsley, chives, chili and garlic whilst stirring.
4. Add in the tomatoes, lemon juice and mussels.
5. Cover the saucepan and cook for 2-3.
6. Remove the saucepan from the heat and take out any mussels which haven't opened and discard them.
7. Serve and eat immediately.

Nutrition:

Calories: 364

Net carbs: 3.3g Fat: 4.9g Fiber: 0.7g

Protein: 8.2g

Roast Balsamic Vegetables

Preparation time: 10 minutes

Cooking time: 45 minutes

Servings: 4

Ingredients:

- 4 tomatoes, chopped 2 red onions, chopped
- 3 sweet potatoes, peeled and chopped
- 100g red chicory (or if unavailable, use yellow)
- 100g kale, finely chopped
- 300g potatoes, peeled and chopped
- 5 stalks of celery, chopped
- 1 bird's-eye chili, de-seeded and finely chopped
- 2g fresh parsley, chopped
- 2gs fresh coriander (cilantro) chopped
- 3 teaspoons olive oil
- 2 teaspoons balsamic vinegar
- 1 teaspoon mustard Sea salt
- Freshly ground black pepper

Directions:

1. Place the olive oil, balsamic, mustard, parsley and coriander (cilantro) into a bowl.
2. Mix well.
3. Toss all the remaining ingredients into the dressing.
4. Season with salt and pepper.
5. Transfer the vegetables to an ovenproof dish
6. And cook in the oven at 200C/400F for 45 minutes.

Nutrition: Calories: 310 Net carbs: 1.1g

Fiber: 0.2g Protein: 0.2g

Tomato and Goat's Pizza

Preparation time: 15 minutes

Cooking time: 20 minutes

Servings: 2

Ingredients:

- 225g buckwheat flour
- 2 teaspoons dried yeast Pinch of salt
- 150mls slightly water 1 teaspoon olive oil
- For the Topping:
- 75g feta cheese, crumbled
- 75g peseta (or tomato paste)
- 1 tomato, sliced 1 red onion, finely chopped
- 25g rocket (arugula) leaves, chopped

Directions:

1. In a bowl, combine all the ingredients for the pizza dough then allow it to stand for at least an hour until it has doubled in size.
2. Roll the dough out to a size to suit you.
3. Spoon the passata onto the base and add the rest of the toppings.

4. Bake in the oven at 200C/400F for 15-20 minutes or until browned at the edges and crispy and serve.

Nutrition:

Calories: 585 Net carbs: 77g Fat: 8.1g

Fiber: 7.6g Protein: 22.9g

Tender Spiced Lamb

Preparation time: 20 minutes

Cooking time: 4 hours 20 minutes

Servings: 8

Ingredients:

- 1.35kg lamb shoulder
- 3 red onions, sliced
- 3 cloves of garlic, crushed
- 1 bird's eye chili, finely chopped
- 1 teaspoon turmeric
- 1 teaspoon ground cumin
- ½ teaspoon ground coriander (cilantro)
- ¼ teaspoon ground cinnamon
- 2 tablespoons olive oil

Directions:

1. In a bowl, combine the chili, garlic and spices with olive oil.
2. Coat the lamb with the spice mixture and marinate it for an hour, or overnight if you can.
3. Heat the remaining oil in a pan, add the lamb and brown it for 3-4 minutes on all sides to seal it.
4. Place the lamb in an ovenproof dish.
5. Add in the red onions and cover the dish with foil.
6. Transfer to the oven and roast at 170C/325F for 4 hours.
7. The lamb should be extremely tender and falling off the bone.

8. Serve with rice or couscous, salad or vegetables.

Nutrition:

Calories: 455 Net carbs: 28g

Fat: 9.8g Fiber: 11g Protein: 20g

Chili Cod Fillets

Preparation time: 10 minutes

Cooking time: 10 minutes

Servings: 4

Ingredients:

- 4 cod fillets each)
- 2 teaspoons fresh parsley, chopped
- 2 bird's-eye chilies (or more if you like it hot)
- 2 cloves of garlic, chopped
- 4 teaspoons olive oil

Directions:

1. Heat a of olive oil in a frying pan, add the fish and cook for 7-8 minutes or until thoroughly cooked, turning once halfway through.
2. Remove and keep warm.
3. Pour the remaining olive oil into the pan and add the chili, chopped garlic and parsley.
4. Warm it thoroughly.
5. Serve the fish onto plates and pour the warm chili oil over it.

Nutrition:

Calories: 246 Net carbs: 5.5g

Fat: 0.5g Fiber: 0.7g Protein: 18.5g

Steak and Mushroom Noodles

Preparation time: 10 minutes

Cooking time: 20 minutes

Servings: 4

Ingredients:

- 100g shitake mushrooms, halved, if large
- 100g chestnut mushrooms, sliced
- 150g udon noodles
- 75g kale, finely chopped
- 75g baby leaf spinach, chopped
- 2 sirloin steaks
- 2 teaspoons miso paste
- 2.5cm piece fresh ginger, finely chopped
- 2 teaspoons olive oil
- 1 star anise
- 1 red chili, finely sliced
- 1 red onion, finely chopped
- 1 fresh coriander (cilantro) chopped
- 1 liter (1½ pints) warm water

Directions:

1. Pour the water into a saucepan and add in the miso, star anise and ginger.
2. Bring it to the boil, reduce the heat and simmer gently.
3. In the meantime, cook the noodles according to their instructions then drain them.
4. Heat the oil in a saucepan, add the steak and cook for around 2-3 minutes on each side (or 1-2 minutes, for rare meat).
5. Remove the meat and set aside.
6. Place the mushrooms, spinach, coriander (cilantro) and kale into the miso broth and cook for 5 minutes.
7. In the meantime, heat the remaining oil in a separate pan and fry the chili and onion for 4 minutes, until softened.
8. Serve the noodles into bowls and pour the soup on top.
9. Thinly slice the steaks and add them to the top.
10. Serve immediately.

Nutrition:

Calories: 296

Net carbs: 24.6g

Fat: 13.7g

Fiber: 0.7g

Protein: 32.9g

Masala Scallops

Preparation time: 10 minutes

Cooking time: 20 minutes

Servings: 4

Ingredients:

- 2 tablespoons olive oil
- 2 jalapenos, chopped
- 1 pound sea scallops
- A pinch of salt and black pepper
- ¼ teaspoon cinnamon powder
- 1 teaspoon garam masala
- 1 teaspoon coriander, ground
- 1 teaspoon cumin, ground
- 2 tablespoons cilantro, chopped

Directions:

1. Heat up a pan with the oil over medium heat, add the jalapenos, cinnamon and the other ingredients except the scallops and cook for 10 minutes.
2. Add the rest of the ingredients, toss, cook for 10 minutes more, divide into bowls and serve.

Nutrition:

Calories: 251

Fat: 4g

Fiber: 4g

Carbs: 11g

Protein: 17g

Tuna and Tomatoes

Preparation time: 5 minutes

Cooking time: 20 minutes

Servings: 4

Ingredients:

- 1 yellow onion, chopped
- 1 tablespoon olive oil
- 1 pound tuna fillets, boneless, skinless and cubed
- 1 cup tomatoes, chopped
- 1 red pepper, chopped
- 1 teaspoon sweet paprika
- 1 tablespoon coriander, chopped

Directions:

1. Heat up a pan with the oil over medium heat, add the onions and the pepper and cook for 5 minutes.
2. Add the fish and the other Ingredient, cook everything for 15 minutes, divide between plates and serve.

Nutrition:

Calories: 215

Fat: 4g

Fiber: 7g

Carbs: 14g

Protein: 7g

Lemongrass and Ginger Mackerel

Preparation time: 10 minutes

Cooking time: 25 minutes

Servings: 4

Ingredients:

- 4 mackerel fillets, skinless and boneless
- 2 tablespoons olive oil
- 1 tablespoon ginger, grated
- 2 lemongrass sticks, chopped
- 2 red chilies, chopped
- Juice of 1 lime
- A handful parsley, chopped

Directions:

1. Combine the mackerel with the oil, ginger and the other ingredients.
2. Toss and bake at 390 degrees F for 25 minutes.
3. Divide everything between plates and serve.

Nutrition:

Calories: 251

Fat: 3g

Fiber: 4g

Carbs: 14g

Protein: 8g

Instant Savory Gigante Beans

Preparation Time: 10-30 Minutes

Cooking Time: 55 Minutes

Servings: 6

Ingredients:

- 1 lb. Gigante Beans soaked overnight
- 1/2 cup olive oil
- One onion sliced
- Two cloves garlic crushed or minced
- One red bell pepper (cut into 1/3-inch pieces)
- Two carrots, sliced

- 1/2 tsp salt and ground black pepper
- Two tomatoes peeled, grated
- 1 Tbsp celery (chopped)
- 1 tbsp tomato paste (or ketchup)
- 3/4 tsp sweet paprika
- 1 tsp oregano
- 1 cup vegetable broth

Directions:

1. Soak Gigante beans overnight.
2. Press the SAUTÉ button on your Instant Pot and heat the oil.
3. Sauté onion, garlic, sweet pepper, carrots with a pinch of salt for 3 - 4 minutes; stir occasionally.
4. Add rinsed Gigante beans into your Instant Pot along with all remaining ingredients and stir well.
5. Latch lid into place and set on the MANUAL setting for 25 minutes.
6. When the beep sounds, quick release the pressure by pressing Cancel and twisting the steam handle to the Venting position.
7. Taste and adjust seasonings to taste.
8. Serve warm or cold.
9. Keep refrigerated.

Nutrition: Calories 502.45 Calories From Fat 173.16 Total Fat 19.63g Saturated Fat 2.86g

Nettle Soup with Rice

Preparation Time: 10-30 Minutes

Cooking Time: 40 Minutes

Servings: 5

Ingredients:

- 3 Tbsp of olive oil
- Two onions finely chopped
- Two cloves garlic finely chopped

- Salt and freshly ground black pepper
- Four medium potatoes cut into cubes
- 1 cup of rice
- 1 Tbsp arrowroot
- 2 cups vegetable broth
- 2 cups of water
- One bunch of young nettle leaves packed
- 1/2 cup fresh parsley finely chopped
- 1 tsp cumin

Directions:

1. Heat olive oil in a large pot.
2. Sauté onion and garlic with a pinch of salt until softened.
3. Add potato, rice and arrowroot; sauté for 2 to 3 minutes.
4. Pour broth and water, stir well, cover and cook over medium heat for about 20 minutes.
5. Cook for about 30 to 45 minutes.
6. Add young nettle leaves, parsley and cumin; stir and cook for 5 to 7 minutes.
7. Move the soup in a blender and blend until combined well.
8. Taste and adjust salt and pepper.
9. Serve hot.

Nutrition: Calories 421.76 Calories from Fat 88.32 Total Fat 9.8g Saturated Fat 1.54g

Okra with Grated Tomatoes (Slow Cooker)

Preparation Time: 10-30 Minutes

Cooking Time: 3 Hours and 10 Minutes

Servings: 4

Ingredients:

- 2 lbs. fresh okra cleaned
- Two onions finely chopped

- Two cloves garlic finely sliced
- Two carrots sliced
- Two ripe tomatoes grated
- 1 cup of water
- 4 Tbsp olive oil
- Salt and ground black pepper
- 1 tbsp fresh parsley finely chopped

Directions:

1. Add okra in your Crock-Pot: sprinkle with a pinch of salt and pepper.
2. Add in chopped onion, garlic, carrotsand grated tomatoes; stir well.
3. Pour water and oil, season with the salt, pepperand give a good stir.
4. Covering and cook on LOW for 2-4 hours or until tender.
5. Open the lid and add fresh parsley; stir.
6. Taste and adjust salt and pepper.
7. Serve hot.

Nutrition: Calories 223.47 Calories from Fat 123.5 Total Fat 14g Saturated Fat 1.96g,

Powerful Spinach and Mustard Leaves Puree

Preparation Time: 10-30 Minutes

Cooking Time: 50 Minutes

Servings: 4

Ingredients:

- 2 Tbsp almond butter
- One onion finely diced
- 2 Tbsp minced garlic
- 1 tsp salt and black pepper (or to taste)
- 1 lb. mustard leaves cleaned rinsed
- 1 lb. frozen spinach thawed
- 1 tsp coriander
- 1 tsp ground cumin
- 1/2 cup almond milk

Directions:

1. Press the SAUTÉ button on your Instant Pot and heat the almond butter.
2. Sauté onion, garlic and a pinch of salt for 2-3 minutes; stir occasionally.
3. Add spinach and the mustard greens and stir for a minute or two.
4. Season with the salt and pepper, corianderand cumin; give a good stir.
5. Lock lid into place and set on the MANUAL setting for 15 minutes.
6. Use Quick Release - turn the valve from sealing to venting to release the pressure.
7. Move mixture to a blender, add almond milk and blend until smooth.
8. Taste and adjust seasonings.
9. Serve.

Nutrition: Calories 180.53 Calories from Fat 82.69 Total Fat 10g Saturated Fat 0.65g

Quinoa and Rice Stuffed Peppers (Oven-Baked)

Preparation Time: 10-30 Minutes

Cooking Time: 35 Minutes

Servings: 8

Ingredients:

- 3/4 cup long-grain rice
- Eight bell peppers (any color)
- 2 Tbsp olive oil
- One onion finely diced
- Two cloves chopped garlic
- One can (11 oz) crushed tomatoes
- 1 tsp cumin
- 1 tsp coriander
- 4 Tbsp ground walnuts
- 2 cups cooked quinoa

- 4 Tbsp chopped parsley
- Salt and ground black pepper to taste

Directions:

1. Preheat oven to 400 F/200 C.
2. Boil rice and drain in a colander.
3. Cut the top stem part of the pepper off, remove the remaining pith and seedsand rinse peppers.
4. Heat oil in a large frying skilletand sauté onion and garlic until soft.
5. Add tomatoes, cumin, ground almonds, salt, pepperand coriander; stir well and simmer for 2 minutes, stirring constantly.
6. Take away from the heat. Combine the rice, quinoaand parsley; stir well.
7. Taste and adjust salt and pepper.
8. Fill the peppers with a mixtureand place peppers cut side-up in a baking dish, drizzle with little oil.
9. Bake for 15 minutes.
10. Serve warm.

Nutrition: Calories 335.69 Calories from Fat 83.63 Total Fat 9.58g Saturated Fat 1.2g

Quinoa and Lentils with Crushed Tomato

Preparation Time: 10-30 Minutes

Cooking Time: 35 Minutes

Servings: 4

Ingredients:

- 4 Tbsp olive oil
- One medium onion, diced
- Two garlic cloves, minced
- Salt and ground black pepper to taste
- One can (15 oz) tomatoes crushed
- 1 cup vegetable broth

- 1/2 cup quinoa, washed and drained
- 1 cup cooked lentils
- 1 tsp chili powder
- 1 tsp cumin

Directions:

1. Heat oil in a pot and sauté the onion and garlic with the pinch of salt until soft.
2. Pour reserved tomatoes and vegetable broth, bring to boiland stir well.
3. Stir in the quinoa, coverand cook for 15 minutes; stir occasionally.
4. Add in lentils, chili powderand cumin; cook for further 5 minutes.
5. Taste and adjust seasonings.
6. Serve immediately.
7. Keep refrigerated in a covered container for 4 - 5 days.

Nutrition: Calories 397.45 Calories from Fat 138.18 Total Fat 15.61g Saturated Fat 2.14g

Silk Tofu Penne with Spinach

Preparation Time: 10-30 Minutes

Cooking Time: 25 Minutes

Servings: 4

Ingredients:

- 1 lb. penne, uncooked
- 12 oz of frozen spinach, thawed
- 1 cup silken tofu mashed
- 1/2 cup soy milk (unsweetened)
- 1/2 cup vegetable broth
- 1 Tbsp white wine vinegar
- 1/2 tsp Italian seasoning
- Salt and ground pepper to taste

Directions:

1. Cook penne pasta; rinse and drain in a colander.

2. Drain spinach well.
3. Place spinach with all remaining ingredients in a blender and beat until smooth.
4. Pour the spinach mixture over pasta.
5. Taste and adjust the salt and pepper.
6. Store pasta in a sealed container in the refrigerator for 3 to 5 days.

Nutrition: Calories 492.8 Calories from Fat

27.06 Total Fat 3.07g, Saturated Fat 0.38g

Slow-Cooked Butter Beans, Okra and Potatoes Stew

Preparation Time: 10-30 Minutes

Cooking Time: 6 Hours and 5 Minutes

Servings: 6

Ingredients:

- 2 cups frozen butter (Lima) beans, thawed
- 1 cup frozen okra, thawed
- Two large russet potatoes cut into cubes
- One can (6 oz) whole-kernel corn, drained
- One large carrot sliced
- One green bell pepper finely chopped
- 1 cup green peas
- 1/2 cup chopped celery
- One medium onion finely chopped
- 2 cups vegetable broth
- Two cans (6 oz) tomato sauce
- 1 cup of water
- 1/2 tsp salt and newly ground black pepper

Directions:

1. Combine the real ingredients in your Slow Cooker; give a good stir.

2. Cover and cook on HIGH for 5 to 6 hours.
3. Taste adjust seasonings and serve hot.

Nutrition: Calories 241.71 Calories from Fat

11.22 Total Fat 1.28g Saturated Fat 0.27g

Soya Minced Stuffed Eggplants

Preparation Time: 10-30 Minutes

Cooking Time: 1 Hour

Servings: 4

Ingredients:

- Two eggplants
- 1/3 cup sesame oil
- One onion finely chopped
- Two garlic cloves minced
- 1 lb. soya mince* see note
- Salt and ground black pepper
- 1/3 cup almond milk
- 2 Tbsp fresh parsley, chopped
- 1/3 cup fresh basil chopped
- 1 tsp fennel powder
- 1 cup of water
- 4 tbsp tomato paste (fresh or canned)

Directions:

1. Rinse and slice the eggplant in half lengthwise.
2. Submerge sliced eggplant into a container with salted water.
3. Soak soya mince in water for 10 to 15 minutes.
4. Preheat oven to 400 F.
5. Rinse eggplant and dry with a clean towel.
6. Heat oil in a large frying skillet, sauté onion and garlic with a pinch of salt until softened.

7. Add drained soya mince and cook over medium heat until cooked through.
8. Add all remaining ingredients (except water and tomato paste) and cook for a further 5 minutes; remove from heat.
9. Scoop out the seed part of each eggplant.
10. Spoon in the filling and arrange stuffed eggplants onto the large baking dish.
11. Dissolve tomato paste into the water and pour evenly over eggplants.
12. Bake for 20 to 25 minutes.
13. Serve warm.

Nutrition: Calories 287.32 Calories from Fat 141.77 Total Fat 16.42g Saturated Fat 2.02g

Red Bean Fricassee

Preparation Time: 10-30 Minutes

Cooking Time: 40 Minutes

Servings: 4

Ingredients:

- 4 Tbsp olive oil
- One onion finely sliced
- Two cloves garlic finely sliced
- Salt and newly ground black pepper
- One can (15 oz) red beans
- One large carrot grated
- 1 1/2 cup vegetable broth
- 1 cup of water
- One can (6 oz) tomato paste
- 1 tsp ground paprika
- 1 tsp parsley

Directions:

1. Heat oil in a large pot and sauté onion and garlic with a pinch of salt until soft.
2. Add red beans together with all remaining ingredients and stir well.

3. In a separate pan, sauté onion and garlic in the olive oil.
4. Reduce heat to mediumand boil for 25 to 30 minutes.
5. Taste and adjust salt and pepper if needed.
6. Serve hot.

Broccoli Stir-Fry with Sesame Seeds

Preparation Time: 10 Minutes

Cooking Time: 8 Minutes

Servings: 4

Ingredients:

- Two tablespoons extra-virgin olive oil (optional)
- One tablespoon grated fresh ginger
- 4 cups broccoli florets
- ¼teaspoon sea salt (optional)
- Two garlic cloves, minced
- Two tablespoons toasted sesame seeds

Directions:

1. Heat the olive oil (if desired) in a large nonstick.
2. Skillet over medium-high heat until shimmering.
3. Fold in the ginger, broccoliand sea salt (if desired).
4. Snd stir-fry for 5 to 7 minutes, or until the broccoli is browned.
5. Cook the garlic until tender, about 30 seconds.
6. Sprinkle with the sesame seeds and serve warm.

Nutrition: calories: 135 fat: 10.9g carbs: 9.7g protein: 4.1g fiber: 3.3g

The Bell Pepper Fiesta

Preparation Time: 10 minutes

Cooking Time: 0 minutes

Servings: 4

Ingredients:

- 2 tablespoons dill, chopped
- 1 yellow onion, chopped
- 1 pound multicolored peppers, cut, halved, seeded and cut into thin strips
- 3 tablespoons organic olive oil
- 2 ½ tablespoons white wine vinegar
- Black pepper to taste

Directions:

1. Take a bowl and mix in sweet pepper, onion, dill, pepper, oil, vinegar.
2. And toss well.
3. Divide between bowls and serve.
4. Enjoy!

Nutrition:

Calories: 120

Fat: 3g

Carbohydrates: 1g

Protein: 6g

Dal with Kale, Red Onions and Buckwheat

Preparation Time: 5 Minutes

Cooking Time: 20 Minutes

Servings: 2

Ingredients:

- 1 teaspoon of extra virgin olive oil
- 1 teaspoon of mustard seeds
- 40g red onions, finely chopped
- 1 clove of garlic, very finely chopped
- 1 teaspoon very finely chopped ginger
- 1 Thai chili, very finely chopped
- 1 teaspoon curry mixture
- 2 teaspoons turmeric
- 300ml vegetable broth
- 40g red lentils
- 50g kale, chopped
- 50ml coconut milk
- 50g buckwheat

Directions:

1. Heat oil in a pan
2. Add the curry powder and 1 teaspoon of turmeric, mix well.
3. Add the vegetable stock, bring to the boil.
4. Add the lentils and cook them for 25 to 30 minutes until they are ready.
5. Then add the kale and coconut milk and simmer for 5 minutes. The Dal is ready.

Nutrition:

- Calories: 289 Cal
- Fat: 18 g
- Carbs: 28 g
- Protein: 13 g
- Fiber: 10 g

Spiced Up Pumpkin Seeds Bowls

Preparation Time: 10 minutes

Cooking Time: 20 minutes

Servings: 4

Ingredients:

- ½ tablespoon chili powder
- ½ teaspoon cayenne
- 2 cups pumpkin seeds
- 2 teaspoons lime juice

Directions:

1. Spread pumpkin seeds over lined baking sheet; add lime juice, cayenne and chili powder.
2. Toss well.
3. Pre-heat your oven to 275 degrees F.
4. Roast in your oven for 20 minutes and transfer to small bowls.
5. Serve and enjoy!

Nutrition:

Calories: 170

Fat: 3g

Carbohydrates: 10g

Protein: 6g

Chicken Salad

Preparation Time: 5 Minutes

Cooking Time: 30 Minutes

Servings: 2

Ingredients:

- ½ red onion, very finely sliced
- 1 tablespoon of sesame seeds
- 150g of cooked chicken-shredded
- Large handful 20g of parsley-chopped
- 100g of baby kale-chopped roughly
- 2 teaspoons of soy sauce
- 1 teaspoon of clear honey
- 1 teaspoon of sesame oil

Directions:

1. Place a frying pan over medium heat.
2. Mix the sesame oil, honey, olive oil, lime juiceand soy sauce to make the dressing.
3. Place the cucumber, red onion, kale, pak choiand parsley in a large bowl and gently mix.
4. Pour the dressing over and mix again.

Nutrition:

Calories: 300 Cal

Fat: 10 g

Carbs: 15 g

Protein: 8 g

Fiber: 0.5 g

Tuna, Egg & Caper Salad

Preparation Time: 5 Minutes

Cooking Time: 20 Minutes

Servings: 2

Ingredients:

- 100g 3½oz red chicory or yellow if not available
- 150g 5oz tinned tuna flakes in brine, drained
- 100g 3 ½ oz. cucumber
- 25g 1oz rocket arugula
- 6 pitted black olives
- 2 hard-boiled eggs, peeled and quartered
- 2 tomatoes, chopped
- 2 tablespoons fresh parsley, chopped
- 1 red onion, chopped
- 1 stalk of celery
- 1 tablespoon capers
- 2 tablespoons garlic vinaigrette see recipe
- 340 calories per serving

Directions:

1. Place the tuna, cucumber, olives, tomatoes, onion, chicory, celeryand parsley and rocket arugula into a bowl.
2. Serve onto plates and scatter the eggs and capers on top.

Nutrition:

Lara Burns

Calories: 310 Cal

Fat: 15 g

Carbs: 14 g

Protein: 0 g

Fiber: 10 g

Mussels in Red Wine Sauce

Preparation Time: 5 Minutes

Cooking Time: 50 Minutes

Servings: 2

Ingredients:

- 800g 2lb mussels
- 2 x 400g 14 oz. tins of chopped tomatoes
- 25g 1oz butter
- 1 tablespoon fresh chives, chopped
- 1 tablespoon fresh parsley, chopped
- 1 bird's-eye chili, finely chopped
- 4 cloves of garlic, crushed
- 400 ml 14fl. oz. red wine
- Juice of 1 lemon

Directions:

1. Heat the butter in a large saucepan and add in the red wine.
2. Reduce the heat and add the parsley, chives, chili and garlic whilst stirring.
3. Add in the tomatoes, lemon juice and mussels.
4. Cover the saucepan and cook for 2-3 minutes.
5. Serve.

Nutrition:

Calories: 364 Cal

Fat: 5 g

Carbs: 26 g

Protein: 16 g

Fiber: 15 g

Roast Vegetables

Preparation Time: 5 Minutes

Cooking Time: 45 Minutes

Servings: 2

Ingredients:

- 4 tomatoes, chopped
- 2 red onions, chopped
- 3 sweet potatoes, peeled and chopped
- 100g 3½ oz. red chicory or if unavailable, use yellow
- 100g 3½ oz. kale, finely chopped
- 300g 11oz potatoes, peeled and chopped
- 5 stalks of celery, chopped
- 1 bird's-eye chili, de-seeded and finely chopped
- 2 tablespoons fresh parsley, chopped
- 2 tablespoons fresh coriander cilantro chopped
- 3 tablespoons olive oil
- 2 tablespoons balsamic vinegar 1 teaspoon mustard
- Sea salt
- Freshly ground black pepper

Directions:

1. Place the olive oil, balsamic, mustard, parsley and coriander cilantro into a bowl.
2. And mix well.
3. Toss all the remaining ingredients into the dressing
4. And season with salt and pepper.
5. Serve.

Nutrition:

Calories: 310 Cal

Fat: 15 g

Carbs: 21 g

Protein: 13 g

Fiber: 10 g

Salmon and Capers

Preparation Time: 10 minutes

Cooking Time: 0

Servings: 4

Ingredients:

- 75g (3oz) Greek yogurt
- 4 salmon fillets, skin removed
- 4 teaspoons Dijon Mustard
- 1 tablespoon capers, chopped
- 2 teaspoons fresh parsley
- Zest of 1 lemon

Directions:

1. In a bowl, mix together the yogurt, mustard, lemon zest, parsley and capers.
2. Thoroughly coat the salmon in the mixture.
3. Place the salmon under a hot grill (broiler).
4. Cook for 3-4 minutes on each side, or until the fish is cooked.
5. Serve with mashed potatoes and vegetables or a large green leafy salad.

Nutrition:

Calories: 321 Cal

Fat: 0 g

Carbs: 0 g

Protein: 0 g

Fiber: 0 g

Rocket salad with Tuna

Preparation Time: 5 minutes

Cooking Time: 15 minutes

Servings: 4

Ingredients:

- 4 slices rustic bread, torn into pieces
- 4 large tomatoes
- 2 Tbsp. olive oil
- 400g tin cannellini beans, drained and rinsed
- ¼ cup Kalamata olives
- 2 cups shredded rocket
- ¼ red onion, sliced finely
- 85g tin tuna

Dressing:

- 2 Tbsp. olive oil
- ½ tsp. dijon mustard
- 1 Tbsp. lemon juice

Directions:

1. Start with setting the oven at 180C.
2. Place the bread slices in braking tray, put olive oil on slices and bake for 10-15 mins.
3. To prepare the dressing mix lemon juice, mustard and oil in a jar.
4. Bring a bowl, add baked bread, onions, beans, tuna, tomatoes and rocket.
5. Put the dressing over salad and enjoy.

Nutrition:

Calories: 338

Carbs: 0g

Fat: 13g

Protein: 0g

Sirt Super Salad

Preparation Time: 5 minutes

Cooking Time: 15 minutes

Servings: 1

Ingredients:

- 1 ounce (50g) arugula
- 3 ounces (100g) smoked salmon slices
- 1 ounce (50g) endive leaves
- 1/2cup (50g) celery including leaves, sliced
- 1/8cups (15g) walnuts, chopped
- 1/2cup (80g) avocado, peeled, stonedand sliced
- 1/8cup (20g) red onion, sliced
- 1 tablespoon extra-virgin olive oil
- 1 tablespoon capers
- 1 large Medjool date, pitted and chopped
- 1/4cup (10g) parsley, chopped
- Juice of 1/4lemon

Directions:

1. Bring a bowl, place large leaves of salad, add all the ingredients one by one in the bowl and stir through the bowl and enjoy.

Nutrition:

Calories: 40

Carbs: 8g

Fat: 0g

Protein: 1g

Strawberry Buckwheat Tabbouleh

Preparation Time: 5 minutes

Cooking Time: 15 minutes

Servings: 1

Ingredients:

- 1/3 cup (50g) buckwheat
- 1/2cup (80g) avocado
- 1 tablespoon ground turmeric
- 1/8 cup (20g) red onion
- 3/8cup (65g) tomato
- 1 tablespoon capers
- 1/8 cup (25g) Medjool dates, pitted
- 2/3cup (100g) strawberries, hulled
- 3/4cup (30g) parsley
- 1 tablespoon extra-virgin olive oil
- 1 ounce (30g) arugula
- Juice of 1/2 lemon

Directions:

1. Start with cooking the buckwheat by mixing the turmeric according to the instructions of package.
2. Drain and let it cool.
3. Now, start chopping the tomatoes, capers, onions, avocados, dates and parsley.
4. Mix all of them with already cooked buckwheat.
5. After that, take the strawberries, slice them and add them in salad.
6. Garnish the salad on the arugula bed.

Nutrition:

Calories: 208

Carbs: 16g

Fat: 11g

Protein: 7g

Fragrant Anise Hotpot Sirtfood

Preparation Time: 2 minutes

Cooking Time: 10 minutes

Servings: 2

Ingredients:

- 1 tbsp. tomato purée
- 1 star anise, crushed (or 1/4 tsp ground anise)
- Small handful (10g) parsley, stalks finely chopped
- Small handful (1Og) coriander, stalks finely chopped
- Juice of 1/2 lime
- 1/2 carrot, peeled and cut into matchsticks
- 500ml chicken stock, fresh or made with 1 cube
- 50g beansprouts
- 1OOg firm tofu, chopped
- 50g broccoli, cut into small florets
- 1OOg raw tiger prawns
- 50g cooked water chestnuts, drained
- 50g rice noodles, cooked according to packet instructions
- 1 tbsp. good-quality miso paste
- 20g sushi ginger, chopped

Directions:

1. Take a pan and put the parsley stalks, lime juice, tomato purée, coriander stalks, star aniseand chicken stock, let them simmer for 10-12 mins.
2. Now add the broccoli, tofu, carrot, water, chestnutsand prawns, gently mix them and let them cook completely.
3. Turn off the heat and add in the miso paste and sushi ginger.
4. Garnish with coriander and parsley leaves and enjoy.

Nutrition:

Calories: 14

Carbs: 3g

Fat: 0g

Protein: 1g

Coronation Chicken Salad Sirtfood

Preparation Time: 2 minutes

Cooking Time: 2 minutes

Servings: 1

Ingredients:

- 75 g Natural yoghurt
- 1 tsp. Coriander, chopped
- Juice of 1/4 of a lemon
- 1/2 tsp. Mild curry powder
- 1 tsp. Ground turmeric
- 6 Walnut halves, finely chopped
- 100 g Cooked chicken breast, cut into bite-sized pieces
- 20 g Red onion, diced
- 1 Bird's eye chili
- 1 Medjool date, finely chopped
- 40 g Rocket, to serve

Directions:

1. Take a bowl, gather the ingredients and mix them in bowland serve the salad on the rocket bedding.

Nutrition:

Calories: 364

Carbs: 45g

Fat: 12g

Protein: 15g

Buckwheat Pasta Salad

Preparation Time: 15 minutes

Cooking Time: 0 minutes

Servings: 1

Ingredients:

- 50g cooked buckwheat pasta
- small handful of basil leaves

- large handful of rockets
- 1/2 avocado, diced
- 1 tbsp. extra virgin olive oil
- 20g pine nuts
- 8 cherry tomatoes, halved
- 10 olives

Directions:

1. Take a bowl or a plate, add in all the ingredients, now scatter the pine nuts all over the ingredients and serve.

Nutrition:

Calories: 220

Carbs: 46g

Fat: 0g

Protein: 8g

Dinner Recipes

Lamb Chops with Kale

Preparation time: 15 minutes

Cooking time: 11 minutes

Servings: 4

Ingredients:

- 1 garlic clove, minced
- 1 tablespoon fresh rosemary leaves, minced
- Salt and ground black pepper, to taste
- 4 lamb loin chops
- 4 cups fresh baby kale

Directions:

1. Preheat the grill to high heat. Grease the grill grate.
2. In a bowl, add the garlic, rosemary, salt and black pepper and mix well.
3. Coat the lamb chops with the herb mixture generously.
4. Place the chops onto the hot side of grill and cook for about 2 minutes per side.
5. Now, move the chops onto the cooler side of the grill and cook for about 6–7 minutes.
6. Divide the kale onto serving plates and top each with 1 chop and serve.

Nutrition:

Calories 301 Total Fat 10.5 g Saturated Fat 3.8 g Cholesterol 128 mg Sodium 176 mg

Total Carbs 7.8 g Fiber 1.4 g Sugar 0 g Protein 41.9 g

Shrimp with Kale

Preparation time: 15 minutes

Cooking time: 10 minutes

Servings: 4

Ingredients:

- 3 tablespoons olive oil
- 1 pound medium shrimp, peeled and deveined
- 1 medium onion, chopped
- 4 garlic cloves, chopped finely
- 1 fresh red chili, sliced
- 1 pound fresh kale, tough ribs removed and chopped
- ¼ cup low-sodium chicken broth

Directions:

1. In a large non-stick pan, heat 1 tablespoon of the oil over medium-high heat and cook the shrimp for around 2 minutes every side.
2. With a slotted spoon, transfer the shrimp onto a plate.
3. In the same pan, heat the 2 tablespoons of oil over medium heat and sauté the garlic and red chili for about 1 minute.
4. Add the kale and broth and cook for about 4–5 minutes, stirring occasionally.
5. Mix in the cooked shrimp and cook for about 1 minute.
6. Serve hot.

Nutrition:

Calories 270 Total Fat 11.9 g Saturated Fat 1.5 g Cholesterol 223 mg

Sodium 312 mg Total Carbs 15.5 g Fiber 2.3 g Sugar 1.2 g Protein 28.3 g

Chicken & Veggies with Buckwheat Noodles

Preparation time: 20 minutes

Cooking time: 25 minutes

Servings: 2

Ingredients:

- ½ cup broccoli florets - ½ cup fresh green beans, trimmed and sliced
- 1 cup fresh kale, chopped and tough ribs removed - 5 ounces buckwheat noodles
- 1 tablespoon coconut oil - 1 brown onion, chopped finely
- 1 (6-ounce) boneless, skinless chicken breast, cubed
- 2 garlic cloves, chopped finely
- 3 tablespoons low-sodium soy sauce

Directions:

1. In a medium pan of the boiling water, add the broccoli and green beans and cook for about 4–5 minutes.
2. Add the kale and cook for about 1–2 minutes.
3. Drain the vegetables and transfer them into a large bowl. Set aside.
4. In another pan of the lightly salted boiling water, cook the soba noodles for about 5 minutes.
5. Drain the noodles well and then rinse under cold running water. Set aside.
6. Meanwhile, in a large wok, melt the coconut oil over medium heat and sauté the onion for about 2–3 minutes.
7. Put the chicken cubes and cook for about 5–6 minutes. Add the garlic, soy sauce and a little splash of water and cook for about 2–3 minutes, stirring frequently.
8. Add the cooked vegetables and noodles and cook for about 1–2 minutes, tossing frequently.
9. Serve hot with the garnishing of sesame seeds.

Nutrition:

Calories 463 Total Fat 11.7 g Saturated Fat 5.9 g Cholesterol 54 mg Sodium 1000 mg

Total Carbs 58.9 g Fiber 7.1 g Sugar 4.6 g Protein 22.5 g

Beef & Kale Salad

Preparation time: 15 minutes

Cooking time: 8 minutes

Servings: 2

Ingredients:

- Steak - 2 teaspoons olive oil - 2 (4-ounce) strip steaks
- Salt and ground black pepper, to taste - Salad - ¼ cup carrot, peeled and shredded
- ¼ cup cucumber, peeled, seededand sliced
- ¼ cup radish, sliced
- ¼ cup cherry tomatoes, halved
- 3 cups fresh kale, tough ribs removed and chopped

Dressing

- 1 tablespoon extra-virgin olive oil
- 1 tablespoon fresh lemon juice
- Salt and ground black pepper, to taste

Directions:

1. For steak: in a large heavy-bottomed wok.
2. Heat the oil over high heat.
3. Cook the steaks with salt and black pepper.
4. Transfer the steaks onto a cutting board for about 5 minutes before slicing.
5. For salad: place all ingredients in a salad bowl and mix.
6. For dressing: place all ingredients in another bowl and beat until well combined.
7. Cut the steaks into desired sized slices against the grain.
8. Place the salad onto each serving plate.
9. Top each plate with steak slices. Drizzle with dressing and serve.

Nutrition:

Calories 262 Total Fat 12 g Saturated Fat 1.6 g Cholesterol 63 mg Sodium 506 mg

Total Carbs 15.2 g Fiber 2.5g Sugar 3.3 g Protein 25.2 g

Prawns with Asparagus

Preparation time: 15 minutes

Cooking time: 13 minutes

Servings: 4

Ingredients:

- 3 tablespoons olive oil
- 1 pound prawns, peeledand deveined
- 1 pound asparagus, trimmed
- Salt and ground black pepper, to taste
- 1 teaspoon garlic, minced
- 1 teaspoon fresh ginger, minced
- 1 tablespoon low-sodium soy sauce
- 2 tablespoons lemon juice

Directions:

1. In a pan, put and heat 2 tablespoons of olive oil in a medium heat and cook the prawns with salt and black pepper for about 3–4 minutes.
2. With a slotted spoon, transfer the prawns into a bowl. Set aside.
3. In the same pan, heat the 1 tablespoon of oil over medium-high heat and cook the asparagus, ginger, garlic, salt and black pepper and sauté for about 6–8 minutes, stirring frequently.
4. Mix in the prawns and soy sauce and cook for about 1 minute.
5. Mix in the lemon juice and remove from the heat.
6. Serve hot.

Nutrition:

Calories 253 Total Fat 12.7 g Saturated Fat 2.2 g Cholesterol 239 mg Sodium 501 mg

Total Carbs 7.1 g Fiber 2.5 g Sugar 2.6 g Protein 28.7 g

Turkey Satay Skewer

Preparation time: 5 minutes

Cooking time: 30 minutes

Servings: 3

Ingredients:

- 250g (9oz) turkey breast, cubed
- 25g (1oz) smooth peanut butter
- 1 clove of garlic, crushed
- ½ small bird's eye chili (or more if you like it hotter), finely chopped
- ½ tsp. ground turmeric
- 200ml (7fl oz.) coconut milk
- 2 tsp. soy sauce

Directions:

1. Combine the coconut milk, peanut butter, turmeric, soy sauce, garlic and chili.
2. Add the turkey pieces to the bowl and stir them until they are completely coated.
3. Push the turkey onto metal skewers.
4. Place the satay skewers on a barbeque or under a hot grill (broiler) and cook for 4-5 minutes per side, until they are thoroughly cooked.

Nutrition:

Calorie: 107 Cal

Fat: 1 g

Carbs: 3 g

Protein: 20 g

Salmon & Capers

Preparation time: 5 minutes

Cooking time: 40 minutes

Servings: 3

Ingredients:

- 75g (3oz) Greek yogurt
- 4 salmon fillets, skin removed
- 4 tsp. Dijon mustard
- 1 tbsp. capers, chopped
- 2 tsp. fresh parsley
- Zest of 1 lemon

Directions:

1. In a bowl, mix the yogurt, mustard, lemon zest, parsley and capers.
2. Thoroughly coat the salmon in the mixture.
3. Place the salmon under a hot grill (broiler).
4. Cook for 3-4 minutes on each side or until the fish is cooked.

5. Serve with mashed potato and green leafy vegetables.

Nutrition:

Calorie: 430 Cal

Fat: 24 g

Carbs: 3 g

Sodium: 860 mg

Protein: 45 g

Chicken Casserole

Preparation time: 5 minutes

Cooking time: 20 minutes

Servings: 3

Ingredients:

- 250g (9oz) tinned chickpeas (garbanzo beans) drained
- 4 chicken breasts, cubed
- 4 Medjool dates halved
- 6 dried apricots, halved
- 1 red onion, sliced
- 1 carrot, chopped
- 1 tsp. ground cumin
- 1 tsp. ground cinnamon
- 1 tsp. ground turmeric
- 1 bird's eye chili, chopped
- 600ml (1 pint) chicken stock (broth)
- 25g (1oz) corn flour
- 60ml (2fl oz.) water
- 2 tbsp. fresh coriander

Directions:

1. Place the chicken, chickpeas (garbanzo beans), onion, carrot, chili, cumin turmeric, cinnamon.
2. And stock (broth) into a large saucepan.
3. Add in the dates and apricots and simmer for 10 minutes.

4. In a cup, stir the corn flour with the water until it becomes a smooth paste.
5. Put the mixture into the saucepan and stir until it thickens.
6. Add in the coriander (cilantro) and mix well.
7. Serve with buckwheat or couscous.

Nutrition:

Calorie: 381.8 kcal Fat: 10.3 g Carbs: 40.6 g Sodium: 2147 mg Protein: 32.3 g

Veal Cabbage Rolls – Smarter with Capers, Garlic and Caraway Seeds

Preparation time: 15 minutes

Cooking time: 40 minutes

Servings: 4

Ingredients:

- 1 kg white cabbage (1 white cabbage)
- Salt
- 2 onions
- 1 clove of garlic
- 3 tbsp. oil
- 700 g veal mince (request from the butcher)
- 40 g escapades (glass; depleted weight)
- 2 eggs
- Pepper
- 1 tsp favorer
- 1 tbsp. paprika powder (sweet)
- 400 ml veal stock
- 125 ml soy cream

Directions:

1. Wash the cabbage and evacuate the outer leaves.
2. Cut out the tail during a wedge.
3. Spot an enormous pot of salted water and warm it to the purpose of boiling.
4. Within the interim, expel 16 leaves from the cabbage during a steady progression, increase the bubbling water and cook for 3-4 minutes.
5. Lift out, flush under running virus water and channel.
6. Spot on a kitchen towel, spread with a subsequent towel and pat dry
7. Cut out the hard, center leaf ribs.
8. Peel and finely cleave onions and garlic.
9. Warmth 1 tablespoon of oil.
10. Braise the onions and garlic until translucent.
11. Let cool during a bowl.
12. Include minced meat, tricks, eggs, salt and pepper and blend everything into a meat player.
13. Put 2 cabbage leaves together and put 1 serving of mince on each leaf.
14. Move up firmly and fasten it with kitchen string.
15. Heat the remainder of the oil during a panand earthy colored the 8 cabbage abounds in it from all sides.
16. Add the caraway and paprika powder— empty veal stock into the pot and warmth to the purpose of boiling.
17. Cover and braise the cabbage turns over medium warmth for 35–40 minutes, turn within the middle.
18. Mix the soy cream into the sauce and let it bubble for a further 5 minutes— season with salt and pepper.
19. Put the cabbage roulades on a plate and present with earthy colored rice or pureed potatoes.

Nutrition:

Calories: 645 kcal

Protein: 182.07 g

Fat: 163.4 g

Carbohydrates: 129.37 g

Fragrant Asian Hotspot

Preparation time: 5 minutes

Cooking time: 15 minutes

Servings: 2

Ingredients:

- 1 tsp. tomato purée
- 1-star anise, crushed (or 1/4 tsp. ground anise)
- Small handful (10g) parsley, stalks finely chopped
- Small handful (1Og) coriander, stalks finely chopped
- Juice of 1/2 lime
- 500ml chicken stock, fresh or made with one cube
- 50g beansprouts
- 50g broccoli, cut into small florets
- 1/2 carrot - 100g raw tiger prawns
- 50g rice noodles
- 100g firm tofu, chopped
- 20g sushi ginger, chopped
- 50g cooked water chestnuts, drained
- 1 tbsp. good-quality miso paste

Directions:

1. In a large saucepan, place the tomato purée, star anise, parsley stalks, coriander stalks, lime juice and chicken stock and bring to simmer for 10 minutes.
2. Add in the carrot, broccoli, prawns, tofu, noodles and water chestnuts and cook gently until the prawns are cooked.
3. Remove from heatand add sushi and miso paste to the ginger.

4. Serve sprinkled with the leaves of the parsley and coriander.

Nutrition:

Calories: 348 kcal Protein: 15.09 g Fat: 9.4 g Carbohydrates: 53.49 g

Tofu Thai Curry

Preparation Time: 5 Minutes

Cooking time: 65 Minutes

Servings: 2

Ingredients:

- 400g (14oz) tofu, diced
- 200g (7oz) sugar snaps peas
- 5cm (2 inches) chunk fresh ginger root, peeled and finely chopped
- 2 red onions, chopped
- 2 cloves of garlic, crushed
- 2 bird's eye chilies
- 2 tablespoons tomato puree
- 1 stalk of lemongrass, inner stalks only
- 1 tablespoon fresh coriander (cilantro), chopped
- 1 teaspoon cumin
- 300mls (½ pint) coconut milk
- 200mls (7fl oz) vegetable stock (broth)
- 1 tablespoon virgin olive oil
- Juice of 1 lime

Directions:

1. Heat the oil in a frying pan, add the onion and cook for 4 minutes.
2. Add in the chilies, cumin, gingerand garlic and cook for 2 minutes.
3. Add the tomato puree, lemongrass, sugar-snap peas, lime juiceand tofu and cook for 2 minutes.

4. Pour in the stock (broth), coconut milk and coriander (cilantro) and simmer for 5 minutes.
5. Serve with brown rice or buckwheat and a handful of rockets (arugula) leaves on the side.

Nutrition:

Calories 346.3.

Total fat 26.4 g.

Saturated fat Trace 2.0 g.

Trans fat 0 g.

Monounsaturated fat 5.4 g.

Cholesterol Trace. 0.0 mg

Beans & Kale Soup

Preparation Time: 15 minutes

Cooking Time: 30 minutes

Servings: 6

Ingredients:

- 2 tablespoons olive oil
- 2 onions, chopped
- 4 garlic cloves, minced
- 1-pound kale, tough ribs removed and chopped
- 2 (14-ounce) cans cannellini beans, rinsed and drained
- 6 cups of water
- Salt and ground black pepper, as required

Directions:

1. In a large pan, heat the oil over medium heat and sauté the onion and garlic for about 4-5 minutes.
2. Add the kale and cook for about 1-2 minutes.

3. Add beans, water, salt and black pepper and bring to a boil.
4. Cook partially covered for about 15-20 minutes.
5. Serve hot.

Nutrition:

Calories 270.4.

Total fat 4.7 g.

Saturated fat Trace 0.6 g.

Trans fat 0 g.

Monounsaturated fat 2.6 g.

Cholesterol Trace. 0.0 mg

Lentils & Greens Soup

Preparation Time: 15 minutes

Cooking Time: 55 minutes

Servings: 6

Ingredients:

- 1 tablespoon olive oil
- 2 carrots, peeled and chopped
- 2 celery stalks, chopped
- 1 medium red onion, chopped
- 3 garlic cloves, minced
- 1½ teaspoon ground cumin
- 1 teaspoon ground turmeric
- ¼ teaspoon red pepper flakes
- 1 (14½-ounce) can diced tomatoes
- 1 cup red lentils, rinsed
- 5½ cups water
- 2 cups fresh mustard greens, chopped
- Salt and ground black pepper, as required
- 2 tablespoons fresh lemon juice

Directions:

1. Heat olive oil in a large pan over medium heat and sauté the carrots, celeryand onion for about 5-6 minutes.
2. Add the garlic and spices and sauté for about 1 minute.
3. Add the tomatoes and cook for about 2-3 minutes.
4. Stir in the lentils and water and bring to a boil.
5. Now, reduce the heat to low and simmer, covered for about 35 minutes.
6. Stir in greens and cook for about 5 minutes.
7. Stir in salt, black pepperand lemon juice and remove from the heat.
8. Serve hot.

Nutrition:

Calories 167.4

Total fat 5.5 g.

Saturated fat Trace 1.2 g.

Trans fat 0 g.

Monounsaturated fat 4.3 g.

Cholesterol Trace. 3.3 mg

Asian Slaw

Preparation Time: 5 Minutes

Cooking time: 25 Minutes

Servings: 2

Ingredients:

- Red cabbage, shredded – 2 cups
- Broccoli florets, chopped – 2 cups
- Carrots, shredded – 1 cup
- Red onion, finely sliced – 1
- Red bell pepper, finely sliced - .5
- Cilantro, chopped - .5 cup
- Sesame seeds – 1 tablespoon
- Peanuts, chopped - .5 cup
- Sriracha – 2 teaspoons
- Rice wine vinegar - .25 cup
- Sesame seed oil - .5 teaspoon
- Sea salt – 1 teaspoon
- Garlic, minced – 1 clove
- Peanut butter, natural – 2 tablespoons
- Extra virgin olive oil – 2 tablespoons
- Tamari sauce – 2 tablespoons
- Ginger, peeled and grated – 2 teaspoons
- Honey – 2 teaspoons
- Black pepper, ground - .25 teaspoon

Directions:

1. In a large salad bowl, toss together the vegetables, cilantroand peanuts.
2. In a smaller bowl, whisk together the remaining ingredients until emulsified. Pour this dressing over the vegetables and toss together until fully coated.
3. Chill the slaw for at least ten minutes so that the flavors meld. Refrigerate the Asian slaw for up to a day in advance for deeper feelings.

Nutrition:

Calories 179

Total fat 11.8 g.

Saturated fat Trace 2.9 g.

Trans fat 0 g.

Monounsaturated fat 4.3 g.

Cholesterol Trace. 3.3 mg

Egg Fried Buckwheat

Preparation Time: 5 Minutes

Cooking time: 45 Minutes

Servings: 2

Ingredients:

- Eggs, beaten – 2

- Extra virgin olive oil – 2 tablespoons, divided
- Onion, diced – 1
- Peas, frozen - .5 cup
- Carrots, finely diced – 2
- Garlic, minced – 2 cloves
- Ginger, grated – 1 teaspoon
- Green onions, thinly sliced – 2
- Tamari sauce – 2 tablespoons
- Sriracha sauce – 2 teaspoons
- Cooked buckwheat groats, cold – 3 cups

Directions:

1. Add half of the olive oil to a large skillet or wok set to medium heat and add in the egg, constantly stirring until it is fully cooked.
2. Remove the egg and transfer it to another dish.
3. Add the remaining olive oil to your wok along with the peas, carrotsand onion.
4. Cook until the carrots and onions are softened, about four minutes.
5. Add in the grated ginger and minced garlic, cooking for an additional minute until fragrant.
6. Add the sriracha sauce, tamari sauce and cooked buckwheat groats to the wok.
7. Continue to cook the buckwheat groats and stir the mixture until the buckwheat is warmed all the way through and the flavors have melded about two minutes.
8. Add the cooked eggs and green onions to the wok, giving it a good toss to combine and serve warm.

Nutrition:

5.68 g of protein.

1.04 g of fat.

33.5 g of carbohydrate.

4.5 g of fiber.

148 milligrams (mg) of potassium.

118 mg of phosphorus.

86 mg of magnesium.

12 mg of calcium.

Aromatic Ginger Turmeric Buckwheat

Preparation Time: 5 Minutes

Cooking time: 65 Minutes

Servings: 2

Ingredients:

- Buckwheat groats rinsed and drained – 1 cup
- Water – 1.75 cup
- Extra virgin olive oil – 1 tablespoon
- Ginger, grated – 1 tablespoon
- Garlic, minced – 3 cloves
- Turmeric root, grated – 1 teaspoon
- Lemon juice – 1 tablespoon
- Sea salt – 1 teaspoon
- Cranberries, dried - .5 cup
- Parsley, chopped - .33 cup
- Pine nuts, toasted - .25 cup (optional)

Directions:

1. Into a medium saucepan, add the buckwheat groats, water, olive oil, ginger, garlic, turmeric, lemon juiceand sea salt.
2. Bring the water in the pot to a boil and then cover the mixture with a lid.
3. Allow it to simmer over medium-low until all of the liquid is absorbed, about twenty minutes.
4. About fifteen minutes into the cooking time of the buckwheat sir, the dried cranberries into the buckwheat allow

them to plump up the last few minutes of the cooking time.

5. Top the buckwheat with the pine nuts and parsley before serving.

Nutrition:

Calories 37

Kale and Corn Succotash

Preparation Time: 5 Minutes

Cooking time: 55 Minutes

Servings: 2

Ingredients:

- Corn kernels – 2 cups
- Black pepper, ground - .5 teaspoon
- Kale, chopped – 2 cups
- Red onion, finely diced – 1
- Garlic, minced – 2 cloves
- Grape tomatoes, sliced in half lengthwise – 1 cup
- Sea salt – 1 teaspoon
- Parsley, chopped – 2 tablespoons
- Extra virgin olive oil – 1 tablespoon

Directions:

1. Into a large skillet pour the olive oil, red onion and the corn kernels, sauteing until hot and tender, about four minutes.
2. Add the sea salt, garlic, kaleand black pepper to the skillet, cooking until the kale has wilted, about three to five minutes.
3. Remove the large skillet from the stove and toss in the parsley and fresh grape tomatoes.
4. Serve warm.

Nutrition:

Calories 137.4.

Total fat 6.7 g.

Saturated fat Trace 1.0 g.

Trans fat 0 g.

Monounsaturated fat 1.8 g.

Cholesterol Trace. 0.0 mg

Asian King Prawn Stir-Fry with Buckwheat Noodles

Preparation Time: 10 Minutes

Cooking Time: 20 Minutes

Servings: 1

Ingredients:

- 150g shelled raw ruler prawns
- 2 tsp. tamari
- 2 tsp. extra virgin olive oil
- 75g soba
- 1 garlic slice
- 1 elevated stew
- 1 tsp. sliced ginger
- 20g red onions
- 40g celery
- 75g green beans
- 50g kcal
- 100ml chicken stock
- 5g celery leaves

Directions:

1. Heat a pan over, at that point cook the prawns in 1 teaspoon of the tamari and 1 teaspoon of the oil for 2–3 minutes.
2. Move the prawns to a plate.
3. Wipe the work out with kitchen paper, as you're going to utilize it once more.
4. Cook the noodles in bubbling water for 5–8 minutes or as coordinated on the parcel.
5. Channel and put in a safe spot.

6. Then, fry the garlic, stew and ginger, red onion, celery, beans and kale in the rest of the oil over a medium – high temperature for 2–3 minutes.
7. Add the stock and bring to the bubble, at that point stew for a moment or two, until the vegetables are cooked yet at the same time crunchy.
8. Include the prawns, noodles and Lovage/celery leaves to the skillet, take back to the bubble at that point expel from the heat and serve.

Nutrition:

Calories 402 Cal

Greek Salad Skewers

Preparation Time: 10 Minutes

Cooking Time: 15 Minutes

Servings: 1

Ingredients:

- 2 wooden sticks, absorbed water for 30 minutes before use
- 8 large dark olives
- 8 cherry tomatoes
- 1 yellow pepper, cut into 8 squares
- ½ red onion, cut down the middle and isolated into 8 pieces
- 100g (about 10cm) cucumber, cut into 4 cuts and divided
- 100g feta, cut into 8 solid shapes
- For the dressing:
- 1 tbsp. extra virgin olive oil
- Juice of ½ lemon
- 1 tsp. balsamic vinegar
- ½ slice garlic, stripped and squashed

Directions:

1. Add leaves basil, finely sliced.

2. Add oregano leaves, finely sliced
3. Liberal flavoring of salt and newly ground dark pepper
4. String each stick with the plate of salad ingredients in the request.
5. Spot all the dressing ingredients in a little bowl and combine altogether.
6. For over the sticks.

Nutrition:

Calories 329 Cal

Sirtfood Couscous

Preparation Time: 10 Minutes

Cooking Time: 20 Minutes

Servings: 1

Ingredients:

- 150g cauliflower, roughly chopped
- 1 garlic clove, finely chopped
- 40g red onion, finely chopped
- 1 bird's eye chilli, finely chopped
- 1 tsp. finely chopped fresh ginger
- 2 tbsp. extra virgin olive oil
- 2 tsp. ground turmeric
- 30g sun dried tomatoes, finely chopped
- 10g parsley
- 150g turkey steak
- 1 tsp. dried sage
- Juice of ½ lemon
- 1 tbsp. capers

Directions:

1. Disintegrate the cauliflower using a food processor.
2. Blend in 1-2 pulses until the cauliflower has a breadcrumb-like consistency.
3. In a skillet, fry garlic, chilli, ginger and red onion in 1 tsp. olive oil.

4. Throw in the turmeric and cauliflower then cook for another 1-2 minutes.
5. Remove from heat and add the tomatoes and roughly half the parsley.
6. Garnish the turkey steak with sage and dress with oil.
7. In a skillet, over medium heat, fry the turkey steak for 5 minutes.
8. Once the steak is cooked add lemon juice, capers and a dash of water.
9. Stir and serve with the couscous.

Nutrition:

Calories 394 Cal

Caramelized Tofu

Preparation Time: 10 Minutes

Cooking Time: 35 Minutes

Servings: 1

Ingredients:

- 1 tbsp. mirin
- 20g miso paste
- 1 * 150g firm tofu
- 40g celery, trimmed
- 35g red onion
- 120g courgette
- 1 bird's eye chilli
- 1 garlic clove, finely chopped
- 1 tsp. finely chopped fresh ginger
- 50g kale, chopped
- 2 tsp. sesame seeds
- 35g buckwheat
- 1 tsp. ground turmeric
- 2 tsp. extra virgin olive oil
- 1 tsp. tamari (or soy sauce)

Directions:

1. Pre-heat your over to 200C or gas mark 6. Cover a tray with baking parchment.
2. Combine the mirin and miso together.
3. Dice the tofu and coat it in the mirin-miso mixture in a resealable plastic bag. Set aside to marinate.
4. Chop the vegetables using a steamer, cook for the kale for 5 minutes and set aside.
5. Disperse the tofu across the lined tray and garnish with sesame seeds.
6. Roast for 20 minutes, or until caramelized.
7. Rinse the buckwheat using running water and a sieve.
8. Add to a pan of boiling water alongside turmeric and cook the buckwheat according to the packet directions.
9. Heat the oil in a skillet over high heat.
10. Toss in the vegetables, herbs and spices then fry for 2-3 minutes.
11. Reduce to a medium heat and fry for a further 5 minutes or until cooked but still crunchy.

Nutrition:

Calories 273 Cal

Stir-fry & Soba

Preparation Time: 10 Minutes

Cooking Time: 25 Minutes

Servings: 2

Ingredients:

- 150g shelled raw king prawns, deveined
- 2 tsp. tamari
- 2 tsp. extra virgin olive oil
- 75 soba
- 1 garlic clove, finely chopped
- 1 bird's eye chilli, finely chopped
- 1 tsp. finely chopped fresh ginger
- 20g red onions, sliced

- 40g celery, trimmed and sliced
- 75g green beans, chopped
- 50g kale, roughly chopped
- 100ml chicken stock

Directions:

1. Warm a skillet over a high heat.
2. And then fry for the pawns in 1 tsp. of the tamari and of olive oil.
3. Transfer the contents of the skillet to a plate.
4. And then wipe the skillet with kitchen towel.
5. Boil water and cook the soba for 8 minutes.
6. Drain and set aside.
7. Using the remaining 1 tsp. olive oil.
8. Fry the remaining ingredients for 3-4 minutes.
9. Add the stock and bring to the boil.
10. Simmering until the vegetables are tender but still have bite.
11. Add the Lovage, noodles and prawn into the skillet.
12. Stir, bring back to the boil and then serve.

Nutrition:

Calories 435 kcal

Mushroom Scramble

Preparation Time: 10 Minutes

Cooking Time: 20 Minutes

Servings: 1

Ingredients:

- 100g tofu, extra firm
- 1 tsp. ground turmeric
- 1 tsp. mild curry powder
- 20g kale, roughly chopped
- 1 tsp. extra virgin olive oil

- 20g red onion, thinly sliced
- 50g mushrooms, thinly sliced
- 5g parsley, finely chopped

Directions:

1. Place 2 sheets of kitchen towel under and on-top of the tofu.
2. Then rest a considerable weight such as saucepan onto the tofu.
3. Ensure it drains off the liquid.
4. Combine the curry powder, turmeric and 1-2 tsp. of water.
5. Using a steamer cook kale for 3-4 minutes.
6. In a skillet, warm oil over a medium heat.
7. Add the chilli, mushrooms and onion, cooking for several.
8. Break the tofu in to small pieces and toss in the skillet.
9. Coat with the spice paste and stir, ensuring everything becomes evenly coated.
10. Cook for up to 5 minutes and fry for 2 more minutes.
11. Garnish with parsley before serving.

Nutrition:

Calories 131 Cal

Fragrant Asian Hotpot

Preparation Time: 10 Minutes

Cooking Time: 15 Minutes

Servings: 2

Ingredients:

- 1 tsp. tomato purée
- 1 star anise, squashed (or 1/4 tsp. ground anise)
- Little bunch (10g) parsley, stalks finely cleaved

- Little bunch (1Og) coriander, stalks finely cleaved
- Juice of 1/2 lime
- 500ml chicken stock, new or made with 1 solid shape
- 1/2 carrot, stripped and cut into matchsticks
- 50g broccoli, cut into little florets
- 50g beansprouts
- 100 g crude tiger prawns
- 100 g firm tofu, slashed
- 50g rice noodles, cooked according to parcel directions.
- 50g cooked water chestnuts, depleted
- 20g sushi ginger, slashed
- 1 tbsp. great quality miso glue

Directions:

1. Spot the tomato purée, star anise, parsley stalks, coriander stalks, lime juice and chicken stock in an enormous container and bring to a stew for 10 minutes.
2. Include the carrot, broccoli, prawns, tofu, noodles and water chestnuts and stew tenderly until the prawns are cooked through.
3. Expel from the warmth and mix in the sushi ginger and miso glue.
4. Serve sprinkled with the parsley and coriander leaves.

Nutrition:

Calories 434 Cal

Greek Skewers

Preparation Time: 15 Minutes

Cooking Time: 30 Minutes

Servings: 2

Ingredients:

- 2 wooden sticks, absorbed water for 30 minutes before use
- 8 enormous dark olives
- 8 cherry tomatoes
- 1 yellow pepper, cut into 8 squares
- ½ red onion, cut down the middle and isolated into 8 pieces
- 100g (about 10cm) cucumber, cut into 4 cuts and divided
- 100g feta, cut into 8 shapes
- For the dressing:
- 1 tbsp. additional virgin olive oil
- Juice of ½ lemon
- 1 tsp. balsamic vinegar
- ½ clove garlic, stripped and squashed
- Scarcely any departs basil, finely hacked
- Leaves oregano, finely slashed
- Liberal flavoring of salt and crisply ground dark pepper

Directions:

1. Thread each stick with the plate of mixed greens ingredients.
2. Place all the dressing ingredients in a little bowl and combine altogether.
3. Pour over the sticks.

Nutrition:

Calories 364 Cal

Sweet-Smelling Chicken Breast with Kale, Red Onion and Salsa

Preparation Time: 15 Minutes

Cooking Time: 35 Minutes

Servings: 2

Ingredients:

- 120g skinless, boneless chicken bosom
- 2 tsp. ground turmeric

- Juice of ¼ lemon
- 1 tbsp. additional virgin olive oil
- 50g kale, slashed
- 20g red onion, cut
- 1 tsp. slashed new ginger
- 50g buckwheat

Directions:

1. To make the salsa, expel the eye from the tomato and slash it finely, taking consideration to keep however much of the fluid as could reasonably be expected.
2. Blend in with the bean stew, tricks, parsley and lemon juice.
3. You could place everything in a blender yet the final product is somewhat different.
4. Warmth the broiler to 220ºC/gas 7.
5. Marinate the chicken bosom in 1 teaspoon of the turmeric, the lemon juice and a little oil.
6. Leave for 5–10 minutes.
7. Warmth an ovenproof griddle until hot, then include the marinated chicken and cook for a moment or so on each side, until pale brilliant, then exchange to the broiler (place on a preparing plate if your skillet isn't ovenproof) for 8–10 minutes or until cooked through.
8. Expel from the broiler, spread with foil and leave to rest for 5 minutes before serving.
9. In the meantime, cook the kale in a steamer for 5 minutes.
10. Fry the red onions and the ginger in a little oil, until delicate however not shaded, then include the cooked kale and fry for one more moment.
11. Cook the buckwheat according to the parcel
12. Add the rest of the teaspoon of turmeric.
13. Serve nearby the chicken, vegetables and salsa.

Nutrition:

Calories 465 Cal

Indian Lentil Soup

Preparation Time: 10 minutes

Cooking Time: 50 minutes

Servings: 2

Ingredients:

- 2 cups of lentils
- 1 small red onion, minced
- 1 stalk of celery, finely chopped
- 1 carrot, chopped
- 2 large leaves of kale, chopped finely, or 1 cup of baby kale, chopped
- 2 sprigs of cilantro, minced
- 3 sprigs of parsley, minced
- ¼-½ chili pepper, deseeded and minced (use more or less to your taste)
- 1 tomato, chopped into small pieces
- 1 chunk of ginger, minced
- 1 clove of garlic, minced
- 5 cups of chicken or vegetable stock
- 1 tsp of turmeric
- 1 tsp extra virgin olive oil
- ½ tsp Salt

Directions:

1. Cook lentils according to the package, removing from heat about 5 minutes before they would be done.
2. In a saucepan, sauté all of the vegetables in the olive oil.
3. Then add the chopped greens last.
4. Then add the ginger, garlic and chili and turmeric powder.

5. Add the stock and simmer for 5 minutes.
6. Add the lentilsand salt.
7. Stir in the precooked lentils and cook longer, on a very low simmer, for 25 more minutes.
8. Remove from the heat and cool.
9. Cut the avocado, remove the pitand slice it, then scoop out the slices just before eating.
10. Top with avocado slice, then serve immediately.

Nutrition:

Energy (calories): 724 kcal; Protein: 78.7 g; Fat: 14.1 g; Carbohydrates: 82.87 g

Shrimp & Arugula Soup

Preparation Time: 5 minutes

Cooking Time: 30 minutes

Servings: 3

Ingredients:

- 10 medium sized shrimp or 5 large prawns, cleaned, deshelled and deveined
- 1 small red onion, sliced very thinly
- 1 cup arugula
- 1 cup baby kale
- 2 large celery stalks, sliced very thinly
- 5 sprigs of parsley, chopped
- 11 cloves of garlic, minced
- 5 cups of chicken or fish or vegetable stock
- 1 tbsp extra virgin olive oil
- Dash of sea salt
- Dash of pepper

Directions:

1. Sauté the vegetables (not the kale or arugula just yet however), in a stock pot, on low heat for about 2 minutes so that they are still tender and still crunchy, but not cooked quite yet.
2. Add the salt and pepper.
3. Clean and chop the shrimp into bite-sized pieces that would be comfortable eating in a soup.
4. Then, add the shrimp to the potand sauté for 10 more minutes on medium-low heat.
5. Make sure the shrimp is cooked thoroughly and is not translucent.
6. When the shrimp seems to be cooked through, add the stock to the pot and cook on medium for about 20 more minutes.
7. Remove from heat and cool before serving.

Nutrition:

Energy (calories): 640 kcal; Protein: 40.05 g; Fat: 16.72 g; Carbohydrates: 85.47 g

Creamy Chicken Soup

Preparation Time: 5 minutes

Cooking Time: 30 minutes

Servings: 3

Ingredients:

- 4 chicken breasts
- 1 carrot, chopped
- 1 cup zucchini, peeled and chopped
- 2 cups cauliflower, broken into florets
- 1 celery rib, chopped
- 1 small onion, chopped
- 5 cups water
- ½ tsp salt
- Black pepper, to taste

Directions:

1. Place chicken breasts, onion, carrot, celery, cauliflower and zucchini in a deep soup pot.
2. Add in salt, black pepper and 5 cups of water.
3. Stir and bring to a boil.
4. Simmer for 30 minutes then remove chicken from the pot and let it cool slightly.
5. Blend soup until completely smooth.
6. Shred or dice the chicken meat, return it back to the pot, stirand serve.

Nutrition:

Energy (calories): 707 kcal; Protein: 82.77 g; Fat: 36.11 g; Carbohydrates: 8.79 g

Broccoli and Chicken Soup

Preparation Time: 5 minutes

Cooking Time: 30 minutes

Servings: 3

Ingredients:

- 4 boneless chicken thighs, diced
- 1 small carrot, chopped
- 1 broccoli head, broken into florets
- 1 garlic clove, chopped
- 1 small onion, chopped
- 4 cups water
- 3 tbsp extra virgin olive oil
- ½ tsp salt
- Black pepper, to taste

Directions:

1. In a deep soup pot, heat olive oil and gently sauté broccoli for 2-3 minutes, stirring occasionally.
2. Add in onion, carrot, chicken and cook, stirring, for 2-3 minutes.

3. Stir in salt, black pepper and water.
4. Bring to a boil.
5. Simmer for 30 minutes then remove from heat and set aside to cool.
6. In a blender or food processor, blend soup until completely smooth.

Nutrition:

Energy (calories): 641 kcal; Protein: 43.04 g; Fat: 48.81 g; Carbohydrates: 4.75 g

Warm Chicken and Avocado Soup

Preparation Time: 5 minutes

Cooking Time: 30 minutes

Servings: 3

Ingredients:

- 2 ripe avocados, peeled and chopped
- 1 cooked chicken breast, shredded
- 1 garlic clove, chopped
- 3 cups chicken broth
- Salt and black pepper, to taste
- Fresh coriander leaves, finely cut, to serve
- ½ cup sour cream, to serve

Directions:

1. Combine avocados, garlic and chicken broth in a blender.
2. Process until smooth and transfer to a saucepan.
3. Add in chicken and cook, stirring, over medium heat until the mixture is hot.
4. Serve topped with sour cream and finely cut coriander leaves

Nutrition:

Energy (calories): 535 kcal; Protein: 43.62 g; Fat: 10.48 g; Carbohydrates: 52.27 g

Healthy Chicken and Oat Soup

Preparation Time: 5 minutes

Cooking Time: 40 minutes

Servings: 3

Ingredients:

- 3 chicken breasts, diced
- 1 small onion, chopped
- 3 garlic cloves
- ½ cup quick-cooking oats
- 1 large carrot, chopped
- 1 red bell pepper, chopped
- 1 celery rib, chopped
- 1 tomato, diced
- 5 cups water
- 1 bay leaf
- 1 tsp salt
- ½ cup fresh parsley leaves, finely cut
- Black pepper, to taste

Directions:

1. Place the chicken, bay leaf, celery, carrot, onion, red pepper, tomato and salt into a soup pot.
2. Add in water and bring to the boil then reduce heat and simmer for 30 minutes.
3. Discard the bay leaf, season with salt and pepper, add in the oats and parsley, simmer for 5 more minutes and serve.

Nutrition:

Energy (calories): 573 kcal; Protein: 63.3 g; Fat: 27.8 g; Carbohydrates: 14.7 g

Asparagus and Chicken Soup

Preparation Time: 5 minutes

Cooking Time: 30 minutes

Servings: 3

Ingredients:

- 2 chicken breast fillets, cooked and diced
- 2-3 leeks, finely cut
- 1 bunch asparagus, trimmed and cut
- 4 cups chicken broth
- 2 tbsp extra virgin olive oil
- ½ cup fresh parsley, finely chopped
- Salt and black pepper, to taste
- Lemon juice, to serve

Directions:

1. Heat the olive oil in a large soup pot.
2. Add in the leeks and gently sauté, stirring, for 2-3 minutes.
3. Add chicken broth, the diced chickenand bring to a boil.
4. Reduce heat and simmer for 15 minutes.
5. Add in asparagus, parsley, salt and black pepperand cook for 5 minutes more.
6. Serve with lemon juice.

Nutrition:

Energy (calories): 623 kcal; Protein: 23.63 g; Fat: 5.48 g; Carbohydrates: 45.27 g

Fish and Quinoa Soup

Preparation Time: 5 minutes

Cooking Time: 40 minutes

Servings: 3

Ingredients:

- 1lb cod fillets, cubed
- 1 onion, chopped
- 3 tomatoes, chopped
- ½ cup quinoa, rinsed
- 1 red pepper, chopped
- 1 carrot, chopped

- ½ cup black olives, pitted and sliced
- 1 garlic clove, crushed
- 3 tbsp extra virgin olive oil
- A pinch of cayenne pepper
- 1 bay leaf
- 1 tsp dried thyme
- 1 tsp dried dill
- ½ tsp pepper
- ½ cup white wine
- 4 cups water
- Salt and black pepper, to taste
- ½ cup fresh parsley, finely cut

Directions:

1. Heat the olive oil over medium heat and sauté the onion, red pepper, garlic and carrot until tender.
2. Stir in the cayenne pepper, bay leaf, herbs, salt and pepper.
3. Add the white wine, water, quinoa and tomatoes and bring to a boil.
4. Reduce heat, coverand cook for 10 minutes.
5. Stir in olives and the fish and cook for another 10 minutes.
6. Stir in parsley and serve hot.

Nutrition:

Energy (calories): 673 kcal; Protein: 42.14 g; Fat: 35.63 g; Carbohydrates: 48.73 g

Bean Stew

Preparation Time: 5 minutes

Cooking Time: 35 minutes

Servings: 3

Ingredients:

- 50g of kale, chopped roughly
- ½ bird's eye chili, chopped finely (optional)

- 40g of buckwheat
- 50g of red onion, chopped finely
- 1 garlic clove, chopped finely
- 1 tbsp of roughly chopped parsley
- 200ml vegetable stock
- 1 tsp of herbes de provence
- 200g of tinned mixed beans
- 1 tsp of tomato purée
- 1 x 400g tin of chopped Italian tomatoes
- 30g celery, trimmed and chopped finely
- 1 tbsp of extra virgin olive oil
- 30g of carrot, peeled and chopped finely

Directions:

1. Heat the oil in a medium sized saucepan placed over medium low heat.
2. Add in the onion, celery, chili, carrot, garlic and herbs (if using) until the onions are soft enough but not coloured.
3. Add the stock, tomato puréeand tomatoes and bring to a boil.
4. Put in the beans and allow for 30 minutes simmering.
5. Add the kales and cook for 5-10 minutes or until the kale is tenderand then add in parsley.
6. As it cools, cook the buckwheat as per the directions on the packet.
7. Drain the buckwheat and serve with the cooked stew.

Nutrition:

Energy (calories): 375 kcal; Protein: 49.82 g; Fat: 13.48 g; Carbohydrates: 33.27 g

Pork with Pak Choi

Preparation Time: 5 minutes

Cooking Time: 40 minutes

Servings: 3

Ingredients:

- 100g of shiitake mushrooms, sliced
- 1 tbsp of corn flour
- 200g pak choi or choi sum-cut into thin slices
- 125ml of chicken stock
- 1 tbsp of tomato purée
- 1 tsp of brown sugar
- 1 clove garlic, peeled and crushed
- 1 shallot, peeled and sliced
- 100g of bean sprouts
- 1 tbsp of water
- 400g of pork mince (10% fat)
- 1 thumb (5cm) fresh ginger -peeled and grated
- 400g of firm tofu, cut into large cubes
- 1 tbsp of rice wine
- 1 tbsp of soy sauce
- A large handful (20g) of parsley, chopped
- 1 tbsp of rapeseed oil

Directions:

1. Place the tofu on kitchen paper, cover it with kitchen paperand then set it aside.
2. In a small bowl, mix water and corn flour and remove the lumps.
3. Add in rice wine, brown sugar, chicken stock, tomato pureeand soy sauce.
4. Also, add in the crushed ginger and garlic them mix.
5. Place a large frying pan or wok on high heat and add oil to it.
6. Add the mushrooms and stir-fry for 2 to 3 minutes until cooked and glossy.
7. Using a slotted spoon, remove the mushrooms from the pan and let them rest.
8. Add tofu to the pan, fry it until it is brown on all sides, remove it with a slotted spoon when done and set aside.
9. Add the pak choi to your pan or wokand stir-fry for about 2 minutes and, then add the mince.
10. Cook it until it cooks through and then add the sauce.
11. Reduce the heat a notch and allow the sauce to bubble around the meat for 1-2 minutes.
12. Add the tofu, beansproutsand mushrooms to the pan and warm them all through.
13. Remove it from the heat and mix in parsley then serve right away.

Nutrition:

Energy (calories): 586 kcal; Protein: 58.47 g; Fat: 32.52 g; Carbohydrates: 19.69 g

Desserts and Snacks Recipes

Once you get through the first week (and I guarantee you it will be a breeze!) you can have one or max. 2 snacks a day if you need to eat something between meals. You can choose to eat an apple or a couple of walnuts. But if you want to satisfy your gourmand side and not just curb your hunger, why don't you try some of these fantastic recipes for snacks or "bites". They can all be prepared in advance and eaten when needed. They also make for fantastic appetizers for your occasional guests. I have included both savory and sweet snacks.

Crunchy potato bites

Preparation time: 10 minutes

Cooking time: 20 minutes

Servings: 2

Ingredients:

- 1 potato, sliced
- 2 bacon slices, already cooked and crumbled
- 1 small avocado, pitted and cubed
- 1 tbsp of extra virgin olive oil

Directions:

1. Spread potato slices on a lined baking sheet.
2. Toss around with the extra virgin olive oil.
3. Insert in the oven at 350 degrees F.
4. Bake for 20 minutes.
5. Arrange on a platter.
6. Top each slice with avocado and crumbled bacon.
7. Serve as a snack.

Dates in a parma ham blanket

Preparation time: 10 minutes

Cooking time: 20 minutes

Servings: 2

Ingredients:

- 12 Medjool dates
- 2 slices of Parma ham, cut into strips

Directions:

1. Wrap each date with a strip of Parma ham. Can be served hot or cold.

Mung beans snack salad

Preparation time: 10 minutes

Cooking time: 20 minutes

Servings: 2

Ingredients:

- 2 cups tomatoes, chopped
- 2 cups cucumber, chopped
- 3 cups mixed greens
- 2 cups mung beans, sprouted
- 2 cups clover sprouts

For the salad dressing:

- 1 tablespoon cumin, ground
- 1 cup dill, chopped
- 4 tablespoons lemon juice
- 1 avocado, pitted, peeled and roughly chopped
- 1 cucumber, roughly chopped

Directions:

1. In a salad bowl.
2. Mix tomatoes with 2 cups cucumber, greens, clover and mung sprouts.
3. In your blender, mix cumin with dill, lemon juice, 1 cucumberand avocado.
4. Blend really well
5. Add the blended cream to your salad, toss welland serve as a snack.

Sprouts and apples snack salad

Preparation time: 10 minutes

Cooking time: 20 minutes

Servings: 2

Ingredients:

- 1 pound Brussels sprouts, shredded
- 1 cup walnuts, chopped
- 1 apple, cored and cubed
- 1 red onion, chopped

For the salad dressing:

- 3 tablespoons red vinegar
- 1 tablespoon mustard
- ½ cup olive oil
- 1 garlic clove, minced
- Black pepper to the taste

Directions:

1. In a salad bowl, mix sprouts with apple, onion and walnuts.

2. In another bowl, mix vinegar with mustard, oil, garlic and pepper and whisk really well.
3. Add the dressing to your salad, toss well and serve as a snack.

Moroccan snack salad

Preparation time: 10 minutes

Cooking time: 20 minutes

Servings: 2

Ingredients:

- 1 bunch radishes, sliced
- 3 cups leeks, chopped
- 1 and ½ cups olives, pitted and sliced
- A pinch of turmeric powder
- Black pepper to the taste
- 2 tablespoons olive oil
- 1 cup cilantro, chopped

Directions:

1. In a bowl, mix radishes with leeks, olives and cilantro.
2. Add black pepper, oil and turmeric, toss to coat and serve as a snack.

Celery snack salad

Preparation time: 10 minutes

Cooking time: 20 minutes

Servings: 2

Ingredients:

- ½ cup raisins
- 4 cups celery, sliced
- ¼ cup parsley, chopped
- ½ cup walnuts, chopped
- Juice of ½ lemon
- 2 tablespoons olive oil
- Salt and black pepper to the taste

Directions:

1. In a salad bowl, mix celery with raisins, walnuts, parsley, lemon juice, oiland black pepper and toss.
2. Divide into small cups and serve as a snack.

Dill and bell peppers snack bowl

Preparation time: 10 minutes

Cooking time: 20 minutes

Servings: 2

Ingredients:

- 2 tablespoons dill, chopped
- 1 yellow onion, chopped
- 1 pound multicolored bell peppers, cut into halves, seeded and cut into thin strips
- 3 tablespoons extra virgin olive oil
- 2 and ½ tablespoons white vinegar
- Black pepper to the taste

Directions:

1. In a salad bowl, mix bell peppers with onion, dill, pepper, oiland vinegar and toss to coat.
2. Divide into small bowls and serve as a snack.

Spicy pumpkin seeds bowl

Preparation time: 10 minutes

Cooking time: 20 minutes

Servings: 2

Ingredients:

- ½ tablespoon chili powder
- ½ teaspoon cayenne pepper
- 2 cups pumpkin seeds

- 2 teaspoons lime juice

Directions:

1. Spread pumpkin seeds on a lined baking sheet.
2. Add lime juice, cayenne and chili powderand toss well.
3. Put it in the oven and roast at 275 degrees F for 20 minutes.
4. Divide into small bowls and serve as a snack.

Apple and pecan bowls

Preparation time: 10 minutes

Cooking time: 20 minutes

Servings: 2

Ingredients: 4 portions

- 4 big apples, cored, peeled and cubed
- 2 teaspoons lemon juice
- ¼ cup pecans, chopped

Directions:

1. In a bowl, mix apples with lemon juiceand pecans and toss.
2. Divide into small bowls and serve as a snack.

Zucchini bowls

Preparation time: 10 minutes

Cooking time: 20 minutes

Servings: 2

Ingredients:

- Cooking spray
- ½ cup dill, chopped
- 1 egg
- ½ cup whole wheat flour
- Black pepper to the taste

- 1 yellow onion, chopped
- 2 garlic cloves, minced
- 3 zucchinis, grated

Directions:

1. In a bowl, mix zucchinis with garlic, onion, flour, pepper, eggand dill and stir well.
2. Shape the mix into 12 portions with the help of small bowls and arrange them on a lined baking sheet.
3. Grease them with some cooking spray and bake at 400 degrees F for 20 minutes, flipping them halfway.
4. Serve at room temperature as snacks.

Cheesy mushrooms

Preparation time: 10 minutes

Cooking time: 20 minutes

Servings: 2

Ingredients:

- 20 white mushroom caps
- 1 garlic clove, minced
- 3 tablespoons parsley, chopped
- 2 yellow onions, chopped
- Black pepper to the taste
- ½ cup low-fat parmesan, grated
- ¼ cup low-fat mozzarella, grated
- A drizzle of olive oil
- 2 tablespoons non-fat yogurt

Directions:

1. Heat up a pan with some oil over medium heat, add garlic and onion, stir, cook for 10 minutes and transfer to a bowl.
2. Add black pepper, garlic, parsley, mozzarella, parmesan and yogurt, stir

well, stuff the mushroom caps with the mix.
3. Arrange them on a lined baking sheet and bake in the oven at 400 degrees F for 20 minutes.
4. Serve them as an appetizer.

Shrimp muffins

Preparation time: 10 minutes

Cooking time: 20 minutes

Servings: 2

Ingredients: 6 portions

- 1 spaghetti squash, peeled and halved
- 2 tablespoons avocado mayonnaise
- 1 cup low-fat mozzarella cheese, shredded
- 8 ounces shrimp, peeled, cooked and chopped
- 1 and ½ cups almond flour
- 1 teaspoon parsley, dried
- 1 garlic clove, minced
- Black pepper to the taste
- Cooking spray

Directions:

1. Arrange the squash on a lined baking sheet.
2. Insert in the oven at 375 degrees F and bake for 30 minutes.
3. Scrape squash flesh into a bowl and add pepper, parsley flakes, flour, shrimp, mayoand mozzarella and stir well.
4. Divide this mix into a muffin tray greased with cooking spray.
5. Bake in the oven at 375 degrees F for 15 minutes.
6. Serve them cold as a snack.

Mozzarella cauliflower bars

Preparation time: 10 minutes

Cooking time: 20 minutes

Servings: 2

Ingredients: 12 portions

- 1 big cauliflower head, riced
- ½ cup low-fat mozzarella cheese, shredded
- ¼ cup egg whites
- 1 teaspoon Italian seasoning
- Black pepper to the taste

Directions:

1. Spread the riced cauliflower on a lined baking sheet and cook in the oven at 375 degrees F for 20 minutes.
2. Transfer to a bowl, add black pepper, cheese, seasoning and egg whites.
3. Stir well, spread into a rectangle pan and press well on the bottom.
4. Introduce in the oven at 375 degrees F and bake for 20 minutes.
5. Let it cool and cut into 12 bars
6. Serve at room temperature as a snack.

Cinnamon apple chips

Preparation time: 10 minutes

Cooking time: 20 minutes

Servings: 2

Ingredients: 4 portions

- Cooking spray
- 2 teaspoons cinnamon powder
- 2 apples, cored and thinly sliced

Directions:

1. Arrange apple slices on a lined baking sheet, spray them with cooking oiland sprinkle cinnamon on it.
2. Put it in the oven and bake at 300 degrees F for 2 hours.
3. Divide into bowls and serve as a snack.

Vegetable and nuts bread loaf

Preparation time: 10 minutes

Cooking time: 20 minutes

Servings: 2

Ingredients: 1 loaf

- 175g (6oz) mushrooms, finely chopped
- 100g (3½ oz) haricot beans
- 100g (3½ oz) walnuts, finely chopped
- 100g (3½ oz) peanuts, finely chopped
- 1 carrot, finely chopped
- 3 sticks celery, finely chopped
- 1 bird's-eye chilli, finely chopped
- 1 red onion, finely chopped
- 1 egg, beaten
- 2 cloves of garlic, chopped
- 2 tablespoons olive oil
- 2 teaspoons turmeric powder
- 2 tablespoons soy sauce
- 4 tablespoons fresh parsley, chopped
- 100mls (3½ fl oz) water
- 60mls (2fl oz) red wine

Directions:

1. Heat the oil in a pan and add the garlic, chili, carrot, celery, onion, mushrooms and turmeric.
2. Cook for 5 minutes.
3. Place the haricot beans in a bowl and stir in the nuts, vegetables, soy sauce, egg, parsley, red wine and water.
4. Grease and line a large loaf tin with greaseproof paper.

5. Let it stand for 10 minutes then turn onto a serving plate.

Mushroom and Tofu Scramble

Preparation time: 10 minutes

Cooking time: 20 minutes

Servings: 2

Ingredients:

- 7 ounces of extra firm tofu
- 2 teaspoon turmeric powder
- 1 teaspoon black pepper
- ounce of kale, roughly chopped
- 2 teaspoons extra virgin olive oil
- ounce of red onion, thinly sliced
- 1 Thai chili, thinly sliced
- 100g mushrooms, thinly sliced
- 4 tablespoons parsley, finely chopped

Directions:

1. Wrap the tofu in paper towels and place something heavy on top to help it drain.
2. Mix the turmeric with a little water until you achieve a light paste.
3. Steam the kale for 2 to 3 minutes.
4. Heat the olive oil in a frying pan over medium heat until hot but not smoking; add the onion, chili and mushrooms and fry for 2 to 3 minutes until they have started to brown and soften.
5. Crumble the tofu into bite-size pieces and add to the pan; pour the turmeric paste over the tofu and mix thoroughly.
6. Add the black pepper and stir.
7. Cook over medium heat for 2 to 3 minutes so the spices are cooked through, and the tofu has started to brown.
8. Add the kale and continue to cook over medium heat for another minute.

9. Finally, add the parsley, mix well and serve.

Nutrition:

123 calories

Apple Pancakes with Blackcurrant Compote

Preparation time: 10 minutes

Cooking time: 20 minutes

Servings: 2

Ingredients:

- 4 ounce of porridge oats
- ounce of plain flour
- 1 tablespoon caster sugar
- ½ teaspoon baking powder
- 1 large green apple, peeled, cored, and cut into small pieces
- 150ml semi-skimmed milk
- I large egg white
- 1 teaspoon light olive oil.
- For the compote:
- an ounce of blackcurrants washed and stalked removed.
- 1 tablespoon caster sugar
- 2 tablespoon water.

Directions:

1. Make the compote first. Place the blackcurrants, sugar and water in a small pan. Bring to a simmer and cook for 10-15 minutes.
2. Place the Oats, flour, baking powder and caster sugar in a large bowl and mix properly.
3. Stir the apple into the powder mixture and then whisk in the milk a little at a time until you have a smooth mixture.

4. Whisk the egg white to a stiff peak and then fold into the pancake batter.
5. Heat ½ teaspoon olive oil in a non-stick frying pan on medium heat and pour ½ of the batter. Reduce heat and allow the pancake to cook properly, flip to the other side with a spatula. Cook both sides until golden brown. Remove and repeat to make 2 pancakes.
6. Serve the pancakes with the blackcurrant compote drizzled over.

Nutrition:

123 calories

Sirtfood Mushroom Scramble Eggs

Preparation time: 10 minutes

Cooking time: 20 minutes

Servings: 1

Ingredients:

- 2 medium eggs
- I teaspoon turmeric
- 1 ounce of kale, roughly chopped
- 1 teaspoon extra virgin olive oil
- 1/2 chili, thinly sliced
- 0.5 ounce of red onions
- Parsley, thinly chopped
- A handful of button mushrooms, thinly sliced

Directions:

1. Steam the kale for 2-3 minutes.
2. Mix the turmeric powder with water to form a light paste.
3. Break into a bowl and whisk, add the turmeric paste, parsley and mix properly.
4. Heat the olive oil in a non-stick frying pan over medium heat and fry the onion, chili and mushroom until they have started to brown and soften.
5. Add the steamed kale to the mixture in the frying pan and stir.
6. Pour the egg mixture into the frying pan and stir.
7. Reduce the heat and allow the egg to cook and stir.

Nutrition:

Calories 156

Protein 54.

Matcha Green Juice

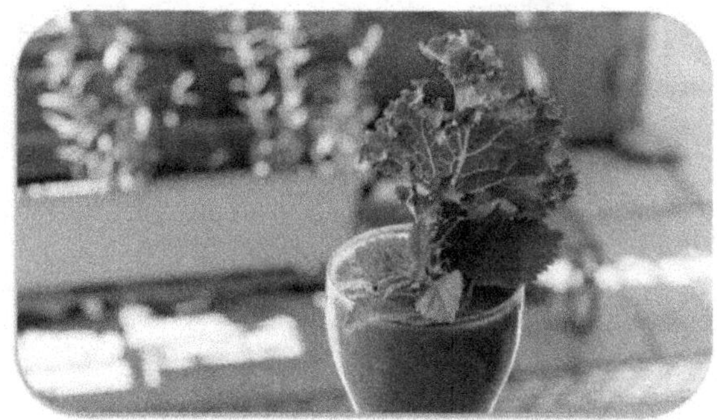

Preparation time: 10 minutes

Cooking time: 0 minutes

Total time: 10 minutes

Servings: 2

Ingredients:

- 5 ounces fresh kale
- 2 ounces fresh arugula
- ¼ cup fresh parsley
- 4 celery stalks
- 1 green apple, cored and chopped
- 1 (1-inch) piece fresh ginger, peeled
- 1 lemon, peeled
- ½ teaspoon matcha green tea

Directions:

1. Add all ingredients into a juicer
2. and extract the juice according to the manufacturer's method.
3. Pour into 2 glasses and serve immediately.

Nutrition:

Calories 113

Celery Juice

Preparation time: 10 minutes

Cooking time: 0 minutes

Servings: 2

Ingredients:

- 8 celery stalks with leaves
- 2 tablespoons fresh ginger, peeled
- 1 lemon, peeled
- ½ cup of filtered water
- Pinch of salt

Instructions

1. Place all the ingredients in a blender and pulse until well combined.
2. Through a fine mesh strainer, strain the juice and transfer into 2 glasses.
3. Serve immediately.

Nutrition:

Calories 32

Kale & Orange Juice

Preparation time: 10 minutes

Cooking time: 0 minutes

Servings: 2

Ingredients:

- 5 large oranges, peeled
- 2 bunches fresh kale

Directions:

1. Add all ingredients into a juicer
2. And extract the juice according to the manufacturer's method.
3. Pour into 2 glasses and serve immediately.

Nutrition:

Calories 315

Cucumber Juice

Preparation time: 10 minutes

Cooking time: 0 minutes

Servings: 2

Ingredients:

- 3 large apples, cored and sliced
- 2 large cucumbers, sliced
- 4 celery stalks
- 1 (1-inch) piece fresh ginger, peeled
- 1 lemon, peeled

Directions:

1. Add all ingredients into a juicer
2. And extract the juice according to the manufacturer's method.
3. Pour into 2 glasses and serve immediately.

Nutrition:

Calories 230.

Fluffy Blueberry Pancakes

Preparation time: 5 minutes

Cooking time: 15 minutes

Servings: 2

Ingredients:

- 1 egg
- 2 oz. self-raising flour
- 1 oz. buckwheat flour
- 1/3 cup skimmed milk
- 1 cup blueberries
- 2 tsp honey

Directions:

1. Mix the flours in a bowl, add the yolk and a bit of mix in a very thick batter. Keep adding the milk bit by bit to avoid lumps.
2. In another bowl, beat the egg white until stiff and then mix it carefully to the batter.
3. Put enough batter to make a 5-inch round pancake to cook 2 minutes per side until done. Repeat until all the pancakes are ready.
4. Put 1 tsp. Honey and ½ cup blueberries on top of each serving.

Nutrition:

Calories: 272, Fat: 4.3g, Carbohydrate: 26.8g, Protein: 23.6g

Banana Strawberry Smoothie

Preparation time: 5 minutes

Servings: 1

Ingredients:

- 1 cup strawberries
- ½ banana
- ½ cup almond milk, unsweetened
- ½ tsp cocoa powder
- 3 cubes ice (optional)

Directions:

1. Blend all ingredients together and serve immediately.

Nutrition: Calories: 92kcal, Fat: 1.3g, Carbohydrate: 12.8g, Protein: 3.6g

Vanilla Parfait with Berries

Preparation time: 5 minutes

Cooking time: 0 minutes

Servings: 1

Ingredients:

- 4 oz. Greek yogurt
- 1 tsp honey or maple syrup
- 1 cup mixed berries, frozen is perfect
- 1 tbsp. buckwheat granola
- ½ tsp Vanilla extract

Directions:

1. Mix yogurt, vanilla extract, and honey. Alternate yogurt and berries in a jar and top with granola.
2. Frozen berries are perfect if the parfait is made in advance because they release their juices in the yogurt.

Nutrition: Calories: 318, Fat: 5.4g, Carbohydrate: 22.8g, Protein: 21.9g

Blueberry Smoothie

Preparation time: 5 minutes

Servings: 1

Ingredients:

- 1 cup blueberries
- ½ banana
- ½ cup orange juice
- 3 cubes ice (optional)

Directions:

1. Blend all ingredients together and serve immediately.

Nutrition: Calories: 87, Fat: 1.1g, Carbohydrate: 11.8g, Protein: 1.6g

Overnight Oats with Strawberries and Chocolate

Preparation time: 5 minutes + 8h

Cooking time: 0 minutes

Servings: 2

Ingredients:

- 2 oz. rolled oats
- 4 oz. almond milk, unsweetened
- 2 tbsp. plain yogurt
- 1 cup strawberries
- 1 tsp honey
- 1 square 85% chocolate

Directions:

1. Mix the oats and the milk and leave overnight.
2. In the morning, top the jar with yogurt, honey, strawberries, and chocolate cut into small pieces.
3. It can be prepared in advance and left up to 3 days in the fridge.

Nutrition:

Calories: 258, Fat: 3.3g, Carbohydrate: 29.8g,

Protein: 13.6g

Chocolate Mousse

Preparation time: 5 minutes

Servings: 1

Ingredients:

- ½ avocado
- 1 tsp cocoa powder
- 1 tsp honey

Directions:

1. Blend all ingredients together and serve immediately.

Nutrition: Calories: 87, Fat: 1.1g, Carbohydrate: 11.8g, Protein: 1.6g

Banana Vanilla Pancake

Preparation time: 10 minutes

Cooking time: 15 minutes

Servings: 2

Ingredients:

- 1 Egg
- 1 Egg White
- 1 Banana
- 2 tsp honey
- 1 cup Rolled Oats
- ¼ tsp Baking Powder
- A pinch of salt
- 1 tsp Vanilla extract
- ½ cup almond milk, unsweetened

Directions:

1. Put half banana, eggs, oats, vanilla, baking powder, salt and almond milk in a blender and blend until smooth.
2. Heat a skillet and, when hot but batter in to form pancakes.
3. Top with honey and the other half banana.

Nutrition: Calories: 232, Fat: 5.3g, Carbohydrate: 22.8g, Protein: 18.6g

Arugula Salad with Turkey and Italian Dressing

Preparation time: 5 minutes

Cooking time: 30 minutes

Servings: 2

Ingredients:

- 8oz. turkey breast
- 1 cup arugula
- 1 cup lettuce
- 2 tsp. Dijon mustard
- 1 tbsp. cumin
- 1/2 cup celery, finely diced
- 2 tsp. oregano
- 1/4 cup scallions, sliced
- 2 tsp. extra virgin olive oil
- Salt and pepper to taste

Directions:

1. Grill the turkey and shred it. Set aside.
2. Mix lettuce and arugula on a plate. Evenly distribute shredded turkey, celery, and scallions.
3. In a small bowl mix all dressing ingredients mustard, oil, lemon juice, oregano, salt and pepper and pour it over the salad just before serving.

Nutrition: Calories: 165 kcal, Fat: 2.9g, Carbohydrate: 13.6g, Protein: 26.1g

Lemon Ginger Shrimp Salad

Preparation time: 15 minutes

Cooking time: 5 minutes

Servings: 2

Ingredients:

- 1 cup chicory leaves
- ½ cup arugula
- ½ cup baby spinach
- 2 tsp. of extra virgin olive oil
- 6 walnuts, chopped
- 1 avocado-peeled, stoned and sliced
- Juice of ½ lemon
- 8 oz. shrimps

- 1 pinch chili

Directions:

1. Mix chicory, baby spinach, and arugula and put them on a large plate.
2. Heat a skillet on medium-high temperature, put 1 tbsp. oil and cook shrimps with garlic, chili, salt, and pepper until they are not transparent anymore (5 minutes)
3. Blend avocado with oil, lemon juice with a pinch of salt and pepper and distribute the dressing on top.
4. Chop the walnuts, put them on the plate as last ingredient and serve.

Nutrition: Calories: 353, Fat: 4.8g, Carbohydrate: 28.1g, Protein: 28.3g

Asian Beef Salad

Preparation time: 15 minutes

Cooking time: 8 minutes

Servings: 2

Ingredients:

- 3 tsp. extra virgin olive oil
- 8 0z. sirloin steaks
- ½ red onion, finely sliced
- ½ cucumber, sliced
- ½ cup cherry tomatoes halved
- 2 cups lettuce
- 1 handful parsley
- 1 tbsp. soy sauce
- ½ bird's eye chili
- 3 tbsp. lemon juice

Directions:

1. Crush the garlic, mix it with finely sliced chili and parsley, 2 tsp olive oil and soy sauce. This will be dressing.

2. Prepare the salad in a bowl placing lettuce on the bottom, then onion, cherry tomatoes and cucumber.
3. Heat a skillet until very hot. Brush the steaks with remaining oil, season them with salt and pepper and cook them to your taste. Transfer the steaks onto a cutting board for 5 minutes before slicing.
4. Drizzle the dressing on the salad and mix well. Place steak slices on top and serve.

Nutrition: Calories 262, Total Fat 12 g, Total Carbs 15.2 g Protein 25.2 g

Avocado Mayo Medley

Preparation time: 5 minutes

Cooking time: 0 minutes

Servings: 3

Ingredients:

- 1 medium avocado, cut into chunks
- ½ teaspoon ground cayenne pepper
- 2 tablespoons fresh cilantro
- ¼ cup olive oil
- ½ cup mayo, low fat and low sodium

Directions:

1. Take a food processor and add avocado, cayenne pepper, lime juice, salt and cilantro.
2. Mix until smooth.
3. Slowly incorporate olive oil, add 1 tablespoon at a time and keep processing between additions.
4. Store and use as needed!

Nutrition:

- Calories: 231
- Fat: 20g
- Carbohydrates: 5g
- Protein: 3g

Amazing Garlic Aioli

Preparation time: 5 minutes

Cooking time: 0 minutes

Servings: 3

Ingredients:

- ½ cup mayonnaise, low fat and low sodium
- 2 garlic cloves, minced
- Juice of 1 lemon
- 1 tablespoon fresh-flat leaf Italian parsley, chopped
- 1 teaspoon chives, chopped
- Salt and pepper to taste

Directions:

1. Add mayonnaise, garlic, parsley, lemon juice, chives and season with salt and pepper.
2. Blend until combined well.
3. Pour into refrigerator and chill for 30 minutes.
4. Serve and use as needed!

Nutrition:

Calories: 813

Fat: 88g

Carbohydrates: 9g

Protein: 2g

Easy Seed Crackers

Preparation time: 10 minutes

Cooking Time: 60 minutes

Ingredients:

- 1 cup boiling water
- 1/3 cup chia seeds
- 1/3 cup sesame seeds
- 1/3 cup pumpkin seeds
- 1/3 cup Flaxseeds
- 1/3 cup sunflower seeds
- 1 tablespoon Psyllium powder
- 1 cup almond flour
- 1 teaspoon salt
- ¼ cup coconut oil, melted

Directions:

1. Preheat your oven to 300 degrees F.
2. Line a cookie sheet with parchment paper and keep it on the side.
3. Add listed ingredients (except coconut oil and water) to food processor and pulse until ground.
4. Transfer to a large mixing bowl and pour melted coconut oil and boiling water, mix.
5. Transfer mix to prepared sheet and spread into a thin layer.
6. Cut dough into crackers and bake for 60 minutes.
7. Cool and serve.
8. Enjoy!

Nutrition:

- Total Carbs: 10.6g
- Fiber: 3g
- Protein: 5g
- Fat: 14.6g

Hearty Almond Crackers

Preparation time: 10 minutes

Cooking Time: 20 minutes

Ingredients:

- 1 cup almond flour
- ¼ teaspoon baking soda
- 1/8 teaspoon black pepper
- 3 tablespoons sesame seeds
- 1 egg, beaten
- Salt and pepper to taste

Directions:

1. Preheat your oven to 350 degrees F.
2. Line two baking sheets with parchment paper and keep them on the side.
3. Divide dough into two balls.
4. Roll out the dough between two pieces of parchment paper.
5. Cut into crackers and transfer them to prepared baking sheet.
6. Bake for 15-20 minutes.
7. Repeat until all the dough has been used up.
8. Leave crackers to cool and serve.
9. Enjoy!

Nutrition:

Total Carbs: 8g

Fiber: 2g

Protein: 9g

Fat: 28g

Black Bean Salsa

Preparation time: 5 minutes

Cooking time: 0 minutes

Servings: 3

Ingredients:

- 1 tablespoon coconut aminos
- ½ teaspoon cumin, ground
- 1 cup canned black beans, no salt
- 1 cup salsa
- 6 cups romaine lettuce, torn
- ½ cup avocado, peeled, pitted and cubed

Directions:

1. Take a bowl and add beans, alongside other ingredients.
2. Toss well and serve.
3. Enjoy!

Nutrition:

Calories: 181

Fat: 5g

Carbohydrates: 14g

Protein: 7g

Corn Spread

Preparation time: 5 minutes

Cooking time: 0 minutes

Servings: 3

Ingredients:

- 30 ounce canned corn, drained
- 2 green onions, chopped
- ½ cup coconut cream
- 1 jalapeno, chopped
- ½ teaspoon chili powder

Directions:

1. Take a pan and add corn, green onions, jalapeno, chili powder, stir well.
2. Bring to a simmer over medium heat and cook for 10 minutes.
3. Let it chill and add coconut cream.
4. Stir well.
5. Serve and enjoy!

Nutrition:

Calories: 192

Fat: 5g

Carbohydrates: 11g

Protein: 8g

Moroccan Leeks Snack

Preparation time: 5 minutes

Cooking time: 0 minutes

Servings: 3

Ingredients:

- 1 bunch radish, sliced
- 3 cups leeks, chopped
- 1 ½ cups olives, pitted and sliced
- Pinch turmeric powder
- 2 tablespoons essential olive oil
- 1 cup cilantro, chopped

Directions:

1. Take a bowl and mix in radishes, leeks, olives and cilantro.
2. Mix well.
3. Season with pepper, oil, turmeric and toss well.
4. Serve and enjoy!

Nutrition:

Calories: 120

Fat: 1g

Carbohydrates: 1g

Protein: 6g

The Bell Pepper Fiesta

Preparation time: 5 minutes

Cooking time: 0 minutes

Servings: 3

Ingredients:

- 2 tablespoons dill, chopped
- 1 yellow onion, chopped
- 1 pound multicolored peppers, cut, halved, seeded and cut into thin strips
- 3 tablespoons organic olive oil

- 2 ½ tablespoons white wine vinegar
- Black pepper to taste

Directions:

1. Take a bowl and mix in sweet pepper, onion, dill, pepper, oil, vinegar and toss well.
2. Divide between bowls and serve.
3. Enjoy!

Nutrition:

Calories: 120

Fat: 3g

Carbohydrates: 1g

Protein: 6g

Spiced Up Pumpkin Seeds Bowls

Preparation time: 5 minutes

Cooking time: 30 minutes

Servings: 3

Ingredients:

- ½ tablespoon chili powder
- ½ teaspoon cayenne
- 2 cups pumpkin seeds
- 2 teaspoons lime juice

Directions:

1. Spread pumpkin seeds over lined baking sheet, add lime juice, cayenne and chili powder.
2. Toss well.
3. Preheat your oven to 275 degrees F.
4. Roast in your oven for 20 minutes and transfer to small bowls.
5. Serve and enjoy!

Nutrition:

- Calories: 170

- Fat: 3g
- Carbohydrates: 10g
- Protein: 6g

Cauliflower Bars

Preparation time: 5 minutes

Cooking time: 30 minutes

Servings: 3

Ingredients:

- 1 cauliflower head, riced
- 12 cup low-fat mozzarella cheese, shredded
- ¼ cup egg whites
- 1 teaspoon Italian dressing, low fat
- Pepper to taste

Directions:

1. Spread cauliflower rice over lined baking sheet.
2. Preheat your oven to 375 degrees F.
3. Roast for 20 minutes.
4. Transfer to bowl and spread pepper, cheese, seasoning, egg whites.
5. And stir well.
6. Spread in a rectangular pan and press.
7. Transfer to oven and cook for 20 minutes more.
8. Serve and enjoy!

Nutrition:

Calories: 140

Fat: 2g

Carbohydrates: 6g

Protein: 6g

Green Juice Recipe

Preparation time: 10 Minutes

Cooking Time: 0 Minutes

Servings 2

Ingredients:

- 1 large handful of rockets
- Two large handfuls of kale
- ½ medium green apple
- Juice of ½ lemon
- ½ level teaspoon of matcha

Directions:

1. Mix the greens well and juice them to get about 50 ml of juice.
2. Juice the apple and the celeryand then peel the lemon and juice it by hand.
3. Pour a little of the juice in a glass, add matcha powderand then stir vigorously. Once it has dissolved, pour it back on the juiceand stir it in. Add some water if the blend is a little too strong for you and serve.

Nutrition: calories 302, fat 8.5, fiber 9.8, carbs 21.8, protein 11.3

Matcha Green Tea Smoothie

Preparation time: 10 Minutes

Cooking Time: 0 Minutes

Servings 2

Ingredients:

- 2 bananas
- 2 tsp Matcha green tea powder
- 1/2 tsp vanilla bean paste or scraped from a vanilla bean pod
- 1 ½ cups milk
- 4-5 ice cubes
- 2 tsp honey

Directions:

1. Add all ingredients except the Matcha to a blender. Blend until smooth. Sprinkle in the Matcha tea powder, stir well or blend a few seconds more or add cooled green tea).

Nutrition: calories 238, fat 9, fiber 5.6, carbs 14.4, protein 8.4

Fruity Granola Bars

Preparation time: 5 minutes

Cooking time: 30 minutes

Servings: 3

Ingredients:

- ¾ cup packed brown sugar
- ½ cup honey
- ¼ cup water
- 1 teaspoon salt
- ½ cup cocoa butter
- 3 cups rolled oats
- 1 cup walnuts, chopped
- 1 cup ground buckwheat
- ¼ cup sesame seeds
- ½ cup dried strawberries or mixed fruits
- ½ cup raisins
- ½ cup Medjool dates, chopped

Directions:

1. In a large pan, combine sugar, cocoa butter, honey, water and salt. Bring to a simmer and cook for 5 minutes.
2. Score deeply into bars roughly 2" wide by 4" tall.
3. Allow to cool for 30 minutes before breaking or cutting along score lines Store in an airtight container.

Nutrition: calories 188, fat 12.8, fiber 9.2 carbs 22.2, protein 16.8

Cardamom Granola Bars

Preparation time: 5 minutes

Cooking time: 30 minutes

Servings: 3

Ingredients:

- 2 cups rolled oats
- ½ cup raisins
- ½ cup walnuts, chopped and toasted
- 1 ½ teaspoons ground cardamom
- 6 tablespoons cocoa butter
- 1/3 cup packed brown sugar
- 3 tablespoons honey
- Coconut oil, for greasing pan

Directions:

1. Preheat oven to 350 degrees F.
2. Line a 9-inch square pan with foil, extending the foil over the sides. Grease the foil with coconut oil.
3. Mix the oats, raisins, walnuts and cardamom in a large bowl.
4. Heat the cocoa butter, brown sugar and honey in a saucepan until the butter melts and begins to bubble.
5. Bake for 30 minutes or until the top is golden brown.
6. Allow to cool for 30 minutes. Using the foil, lift the granola out of the pan and place on cutting board.
7. Cut into 18 bars.

Nutrition: calories 232, fat 5.5, fiber 7.5, carbs 20.9, protein 16.8

Coconut Brownie Bites

Preparation time: 5 minutes

Cooking time: 40 minutes

Servings: 3

Ingredients:

- ¼ cup unsweetened cocoa powder
- ¼ cup unsweetened desiccated or shredded coconut

Directions:

1. Place everything in a food processor and blend until well combined.
2. Roll into 1" balls.
3. Roll balls in coconut until well-covered and place on wax paper lined baking sheet.
4. Freeze for 30 minutes or refrigerate for up to 2 hours.

Nutrition: calories 282, fat 11.5, fiber 5.5, carbs 17.9, protein 14.8

Kale & Fruit Juice

Preparation Time: 10 minutes

Cooking Time: 10 minutes

Servings: 2

Ingredients:

- 2 large green apples, cored and sliced
- Large pears, cored and sliced
- 3 cups fresh kale leaves
- 3 celery stalks
- 1 lemon, peeled

Directions:

1. Add all ingredients into a juicer
2. and extract the juice according to the manufacturer's method.
3. Pour into 2 glasses and serve immediately.

Nutrition:

Calories 293, Fat 0.8 g, Carbs 74.6 g, Protein 4.6 g, Sodium 69 mg

Kale, Carrot, & Grapefruit Juice

Preparation Time: 10 minutes

Cooking Time: 10 minutes

Servings: 2

Ingredients:

- 3 cups fresh kale
- 2 large Granny Smith apples, cored and sliced
- 2 medium carrots, peeled and chopped
- 2 medium grapefruit, peeled
- 1 teaspoon fresh lemon juice

Directions:

1. Add all ingredients into a juicer.
2. and extract the juice according to the manufacturer's method.
3. Pour into 2 glasses and serve immediately.

Nutrition: Calories 232 g, Fat 0.6g, Carbs 57.7g, Protein 4.9g, Sodium 88mg

Buckwheat Granola

Preparation Time: 15 minutes

Cooking Time: 30 minutes

Servings: 10

Ingredients:

- 2 cups raw buckwheat groats
- ¾ cup pumpkin seeds
- ¾ cup almonds, chopped
- 1 cup unsweetened coconut flakes
- 1 teaspoon ground cinnamon
- 1 teaspoon ground ginger
- 1 ripe banana, peeled
- 2 tablespoons maple syrup
- 2 tablespoons olive oil

Directions:

1. Preheat your oven to 350ºF. In a bowl, place the buckwheat groats, coconut flakes, pumpkin seeds, almonds and spices and mix well.
2. In another bowl, add the banana and with a fork, mash well.
3. Add to the buckwheat mixture maple syrup and oil and mix until well combined.
4. Transfer the mixture onto the prepared baking sheet and spread in an even layer. Bake for about 25–30 minutes, stirring once halfway through.
5. Remove the baking sheet from oven and set aside to cool.

Nutrition: Calories 252, Fat 14.3 g, Carbs 27.6 g,

Apple Pancakes

Preparation Time: 15 minutes

Cooking Time: 24 minutes

Servings: 6

Ingredients:

- ½ cup buckwheat flour
- 2 tablespoons coconut sugar
- 1 teaspoon baking powder
- ½ teaspoon ground cinnamon
- 1/3 cup unsweetened almond milk
- 1 egg, beaten lightly
- 2 granny smith apples, peeled, coredand grated

Directions:

1. In a bowl, place the flour, coconut sugarand cinnamonand mix well.
2. In another bowl, place the almond milk and egg and beat until well combined.
3. Now, place the flour mixture and mix until well combined.

4. Fold in the grated apples.
5. Heat a lightly greased non-stick wok over medium-high heat.
6. Add desired amount of mixture and with a spoon, spread into an even layer.
7. Cook for 1–2 minutes on each side.
8. Repeat with the remaining mixture.
9. Serve warm with the drizzling of honey.

Nutrition: Calories 93, Fat 21g, Carbs 22g, Protein 25g, Sodium 23mg

Matcha Pancakes

Preparation Time: 15 minutes

Cooking Time: 24 minutes

Servings: 6

Ingredients:

- 2 tablespoons flax meal
- 5 tablespoons warm water
- 1 cup spelt flour
- 1 cup buckwheat flour
- 1 tablespoon matcha powder
- 1 tablespoon baking powder
- Pinch of salt
- ¾ cup unsweetened almond milk
- 1 tablespoon olive oil
- 1/3 cup raw honey

Directions:

1. In a bowl, add the flax meal and warm water and mix well. Set aside for about 5 minutes.
2. In another bowl, place the flours, matcha powder, baking powder and salt and mix well.
3. In the bowl of flax meal mixture, place the almond milk, oil and vanilla extract and beat until well combined.

4. Now, place the flour mixture and mix until a smooth textured mixture is formed.
5. Heat a lightly greased non-stick wok over medium-high heat.
6. Add desired amount of mixture and with a spoon, spread into an even layer.
7. Cook for about 2–3 minutes.
8. Carefully, flip the side and cook for about 1 minute.
9. Repeat with the remaining mixture.
10. Serve warm with the drizzling of honey.

Nutrition: Calories 232, Fat 4.6g, Carbs 46.3 g

Smoked Salmon & Kale Scramble

Preparation Time: 10 minutes

Cooking Time: 9 minutes

Servings: 3

Ingredients:

- 2 cups fresh kale, tough ribs removed and chopped finely
- 1 tablespoon coconut oil
- Ground black pepper, to taste
- ½ cup smoked salmon, crumbled
- 4 eggs, beaten

Directions:

1. In a wok, melt the coconut oil over high heat and cook the kale with black pepper for about 3–4 minutes.
2. Stir in the smoked salmon and reduce the heat to medium.
3. Add the eggs and cook for about 3–4 minutes, stirring frequently.
4. Serve immediately.

Nutrition: Calories 257, Fat 17g, Carbs 7.7g, Protein 19.3 g, Sodium 419 mg

Kale & Mushroom Frittata

Preparation Time: 15 minutes

Cooking Time: 30 minutes

Servings: 5

Ingredients:

- 8 eggs
- ½ cup unsweetened almond milk
- Salt and ground black pepper, to taste
- 1 tablespoon olive oil
- 1 onion, chopped
- 1 garlic clove, minced
- 1 cup fresh mushrooms, chopped
- 1½ cups fresh kale, tough ribs removed and chopped

Directions:

1. Preheat oven to 350ºF.
2. In a large bowl, place the eggs, coconut milk, salt and black pepper.
3. and beat well. Set aside.
4. In a large ovenproof wok, heat the oil over medium heat.
5. and sauté the onion and garlic for about 3–4 minutes.
6. Add the squash, kale, bell pepper, salt and black pepper.
7. and cook for about 8–10 minutes.
8. Stir in the mushrooms and cook for about 3–4 minutes.
9. Add the kale and cook for about 5 minutes.
10. Place the egg mixture on top evenly.
11. and cook for about 4 minutes, without stirring.
12. Transfer the wok in the oven.
13. and bake for about 12–15 minutes or until desired doneness.
14. Remove from the oven.
15. and place the frittata side for about 3–5 minutes before serving.
16. Cut into desired sized wedges and serve.

Nutrition: Calories 151, Fat 10.2g, Protein 10.3g, Sodium 156 mg

Kale, Apple, & Cranberry Salad

Preparation Time: 15 minutes

Cooking Time: 15 minutes

Servings: 4

Ingredients:

- 6 cups fresh baby kale
- 3 large apples, cored and sliced
- ¼ cup unsweetened dried cranberries
- ¼ cup almonds, sliced
- 2 tablespoons extra-virgin olive oil
- 1 tablespoon raw honey
- Salt and ground black pepper, to taste

Directions:

1. In a salad bowl, place all the ingredients and toss to coat well.
2. Serve immediately.

Nutrition: Calories 253. Fat 10.3g, Carbs 40.7g, Protein 4.7 g, Sodium 84mg

Arugula, Strawberry, & Orange Salad

Preparation Time: 15 minutes

Cooking Time: 15 minutes

Servings: 4

Ingredients:

- Salad
- 6 cups fresh baby arugula
- 1½ cups fresh strawberries, hulled and sliced

- 2 oranges, peeled and segmented
- Dressing
- 2 tablespoons fresh lemon juice
- 1 tablespoon raw honey
- 2 teaspoons extra-virgin olive oil
- 1 teaspoon Dijon mustard
- Salt and ground black pepper, to taste

Directions:

1. For salad: in a salad bowl, place all ingredients and mix.
2. For dressing: place all ingredients in another bowl and beat until well combined.
3. Place dressing on top of salad and toss to coat well.
4. Serve immediately.

Nutrition: Calories 107, Fat 2.9g, Carbs 20.6g,

Protein 2.1g, Sodium 63 mg

Beef & Kale Salad

Preparation Time: 15 minutes

Cooking Time: 8 minutes

Servings: 2

Ingredients:

- For Steak
- 2 teaspoons olive oil
- 2 (4-ounce) strip steaks
- Salt and ground black pepper, to taste
- Salad
- ¼ cup carrot, peeled and shredded
- ¼ cup cucumber, peeled, seededand sliced
- ¼ cup radish, sliced
- ¼ cup cherry tomatoes, halved
- 3 cups fresh kale, tough ribs removed and chopped
- For Dressing

- 1 tablespoon extra-virgin olive oil
- 1 tablespoon fresh lemon juice
- Salt and ground black pepper, to taste

Directions:

1. For steak: in a large heavy-bottomed wok.
2. Heat the oil over high heat.
3. Cook the steaks with salt and black pepper for about 3–4 minutes per side.
4. Transfer the steaks onto a cutting board for about 5 minutes before slicing.
5. For salad: place all ingredients in a salad bowl and mix.
6. For dressing: place all ingredients in another bowl and beat until well combined.
7. Cut the steaks into desired sized slices against the grain.
8. Place the salad onto each serving plate.
9. Top each plate with steak slices.
10. Drizzle with dressing and serve.

Nutrition: Calories 262, Fat 12g, Protein 25.2g, Sodium 506 mg

Salmon Burgers

Preparation Time: 20 minutes

Cooking Time: 15 minutes

Servings: 5

Ingredients:

- For Burgers
- 1 teaspoon olive oil
- 1 cup fresh kale, tough ribs removed and chopped
- 1/3 cup shallots, chopped finely
- Salt and ground black pepper, to taste
- 16 ounces skinless salmon fillets
- ¾ cup cooked quinoa
- 2 tablespoons Dijon mustard

- 1 large egg, beaten
- For Salad
- 2½ tablespoons olive oil
- 2½ tablespoons red wine vinegar
- Salt and ground black pepper, to taste
- 8 cups fresh baby arugula
- 2 cups cherry tomatoes, halved

Directions:

1. For burgers: in a large non-stick wok, heat the oil over medium heat and sauté the kale, shallots, salt and black pepper for about 4–5 minutes.
2. Remove from heat and transfer the kale mixture into a large bowl.
3. Set aside to cool slightly.
4. With a knife, chop 4 ounces of salmon and transfer into the bowl of kale mixture.
5. In a food processor, add the remaining salmon and pulse until finely chopped.
6. Transfer the finely chopped salmon into the bowl of kale mixture.
7. Then, add remaining ingredients and stir until fully combined.
8. Make 5 equal-sized patties from the mixture.
9. Heat a lightly greased large non-stick wok over medium heat and cook the patties for about 4–5 minutes per side.
10. For dressing: in a glass bowl, add the oil, vinegar, shallots, salt and black pepperand beat until well combined.
11. Add arugula and tomatoes and toss to coat well.
12. Divide the salad onto on serving plates and top each with 1 patty.
13. Serve immediately.

Nutrition: Calories 329, Fat 15.8g, Carbs 24g, Protein 24.9g, Sodium 177 mg

Chicken with Broccoli & Mushrooms

Preparation Time: 15 minutes

Cooking Time: 25 minutes

Servings: 6

Ingredients:

- 3 tablespoons olive oil
- 1-pound skinless, boneless chicken breast, cubed
- 1 medium onion, chopped
- 6 garlic cloves, minced
- 2 cups fresh mushrooms, sliced
- 16 ounces small broccoli florets
- ¼ cup water
- Salt and ground black pepper, to taste

Directions:

1. Heat the oil in a large wok over medium heat and cook the chicken cubes for about 4–5 minutes.
2. With a slotted spoon, transfer the chicken cubes onto a plate.
3. In the same wok, add the onion and sauté for about 4–5 minutes.
4. Add the mushrooms and cook for about 4–5 minutes.
5. Stir in the cooked chicken, broccoli and water and cook (covered) for about 8–10 minutes, stirring occasionally.
6. Stir in salt and black pepper and remove from heat.
7. Serve hot.

Nutrition: Calories 197, Fat 10.1 g, Carbs 8.5g; Protein20.1g, Sodium 82mg

Lemon Ricotta Cookies with Lemon Glaze

Preparation Time: 10 Minutes

Cooking Time: 15 Minutes

Servings: 10

Ingredients:

- 2 ½ cups all-purpose flour
- 1 tsp. baking powder
- 1 tsp. salt
- 1 tbsp. unsalted butter softened
- 2 cups of sugar
- 2 eggs
- 1 teaspoon (15-ounces) container whole-milk ricotta cheese
- 3 tbsp. lemon juice
- zest of one lemon

Glaze:

- 11/2 cups powdered sugar
- 3 tbsp. lemon juice
- zest of one lemon

Directions:

1. Preheat the oven to 375 degrees f.
2. Prepare a medium bowl; combine the flour, baking powder and salt. Set-aside.
3. From the big bowl, blend the butter and the sugar. With an electric mixer, beat the sugar and butter until light and fluffy, about three minutes. Then add eggs one at a time, beating until incorporated.
4. Insert the ricotta cheese, lemon juice and lemon zest. Beat to blend. Stir in the dry ingredients.
5. Line two baking sheets with parchment paper. Spoon the dough (approximately 2 tablespoons of each cookie) on the prepared baking sheets.
6. Then bake for 15 minutes or until slightly golden at the borders. Remove from the oven and allow the cookies to remain on the baking sheet for about 20 minutes.

7. For Glaze: combine the powdered sugar, lemon juice and lemon zest in a small bowl and then stir until smooth. Spoon approximately 1/2-tsp on each cookie and use of the back of the spoon to disperse lightly. Allow glaze to harden for approximately two hours. Pack the biscuits in a decorative jar.

Nutrition:

Calories: 360 Cal

Fat: 2.5 g

Carbs: 82.3 g

Fiber: 0.9 g

Protein: 4.5 g

Dark Chocolate Pretzel Cookies

Preparation Time: 20 Minutes

Cooking Time: 25 Minutes

Servings: 4

Ingredients:

- 1 cup yogurt
- 1/2 tsp. baking soda
- 1/4 teaspoon of salt
- 1/4 tsp. cinnamon
- 4 tbsp. butter (softened/0
- 1/3 cup brown sugar
- 1 egg
- 1/2 tsp. vanilla
- 1/2 cup dark chocolate chips
- 1/2 cup pretzels, chopped

Directions:

1. Preheat the oven to 350 degrees.
2. First, whisk together the butter, sugar, vanilla and egg in a medium mixing bowl.

3. In a separate bowl, place and stir together the salt, baking soda and flour.
4. Stir the bread mixture in, using all the wet components, along with the chocolate chips and pretzels until just blended.
5. Drop a large spoonful of dough on a baking sheet (unlined).
6. Bake for 15-17 minutes, or until the bottoms are somewhat all crispy.
7. Allow cooling on a wire rack.

Nutrition:

Calories: 392 Cal

Fat: 18.2 g

Carbs: 50.2 g

Fiber: 1 g

Protein: 9.1 g

Mascarpone Cheesecake with Almond Crust

Preparation Time: 5 Minutes

Cooking Time: 10 Minutes

Servings: 4

Ingredients:

Crust:

- 1/2 cup slivered almonds
- 8 tsp. - or 2/3 cup graham cracker crumbs
- 2 tbsp. sugar
- 1 tbsp. salted butter melted

Filling:

- 1 (8-ounces) packages cream cheese, room temperature
- 1 (8-ounces) container mascarpone cheese, room temperature
- 3/4 cup sugar

- 1 tsp. fresh lemon juice (I needed to use imitation lemon-juice)
- 1 tsp. vanilla extract
- 2 large eggs, room temperature

Directions:

For the crust:

1. First, preheat oven to 350 degrees F. You will need a 9-inch pan (I had a throw off). Finely grind the almonds, cracker crumbs sugar in a food processor (I used my Magical Bullet). Then add the butter and process until moist crumbs form.
2. Press the almond mixture on the base of the prepared pan (maybe not on the edges of the pan). Bake the crust until its set and start to brown, about 1-2 minutes. Cool. Reduce the oven temperature to 325 degrees F.
3. For your filling: with an electric mixer, beat the cream cheese, mascarpone cheese and sugar in a large bowl until smooth, occasionally scraping down the sides of the jar using a rubber spatula. Beat in the lemon juice and vanilla. Add the eggs one at a time and beat until combined after each addition.
4. Pour the cheese mixture on the crust from the pan. Put the pan into a big skillet or Pyrex dish pour enough hot water to the roasting pan to come halfway up the sides of one's skillet. Bake until the middle of the filling moves slightly when the pan is gently shaken, about 1 hour (the dessert will get hard when it's cold). Transfer the cake to a stand; cool for 1 hour. Refrigerate until the cheesecake is cold, at least eight hours.
5. Topping: squeeze just a small thick cream in the microwave using a chopped Lindt dark chocolate

afterward, get a Ziplock baggie and cut out a hole at the corner, then pour the melted chocolate into the baggie and used this to decorate the cake!

Nutrition:

Calories: 550 Cal

Fat: 40.7 g

Carbs: 36.9 g

Fiber: 3.5 g

Protein: 11.5 g

Home-made Ice Cream Drumsticks

Preparation Time: 20 Minutes

Cooking Time: 0 Minutes

Servings: 4

Ingredients:

- Vanilla ice cream
- Two Lindt hazelnut chunks
- Magical shell - out chocolate
- Sugar levels
- Nuts (I mixed crushed peppers and unsalted peanuts)
- Parchment paper

Directions:

1. Soften ice cream and mixing topping - I had two sliced Lindt hazelnut balls.
2. Fill underside of Magic shell with sugar and nuts and top with ice-cream.
3. Wrap parchment paper round cone and then fill cone over about 1.5 inches across the cap of the cone (the paper can help to carry its shape).
4. Sprinkle with magical nuts and shells.
5. Freeze for about 20 minutes before the ice cream is eaten.

Nutrition:

Calories: 419 Cal

Fat: 18.6 g

Carbs: 63.6 g

Fiber: 2.9 g

Protein: 5 g

Peach and Blueberry Pie

Preparation Time: 10 Minutes

Cooking Time: 40 Minutes

Servings: 16

Ingredients:

- 1 box of noodle dough
- Filling:
- 5 peaches, peeled and chopped (I used roasted peaches)
- 3 cups strawberries
- 3/4 cup sugar
- 1/4 cup bread
- Juice of 1/2 lemon
- 1 egg yolk, beaten

Directions:

1. Preheat oven to 400 degrees.
2. Place dough to a 9-inch pie plate
3. In a big bowl, combine tomatoes, sugar, bread and lemon juice, then toss to combine. Pour into the pie plate, mounding at the center.
4. Simply take some bread and then cut into bits, then put a pie shirt and put the dough in addition to pressing on edges.
5. Brush crust with egg wash then sprinkles with sugar.
6. Set onto a parchment paper-lined baking sheet.
7. Bake at 400 for about 20 minutes, until crust is browned at borders.

8. Turn oven down to 350, bake for another 40 minutes.
9. Remove and let sit at least 30 minutes.
10. Have with vanilla ice-cream.

Nutrition:

Calories: 80 Cal

Fat: 1.1 g

Carbs: 17.8 g

Fiber: 1.3 g

Protein: 1.1 g

Pear, Cranberry and Chocolate Crisp

Preparation Time: 15 Minutes

Cooking Time: 10 Minutes

Servings: 10

Ingredients:

- 1/2 cup flour
- 1/2 cup brown sugar
- 1 tsp. cinnamon
- 1/8 tsp. salt
- 3/4 cup yogurt
- 1/4 cup sliced peppers
- 1/3 cup butter, melted
- 1 teaspoon vanilla

Filling:

- 1 tbsp. brown sugar
- 1/4 cup dried cranberries
- 1 teaspoon of lemon juice
- Two handfuls of milk chocolate chips

Directions:

1. Preheat oven to 375.
2. Spray a casserole dish with a butter spray.
3. Put all of the topping ingredients: flour, sugar, cinnamon, salt, nuts, etc.

4. Butter a bowl and then mix. Set aside.
5. In a large bowl, combine the sugar, lemon juice, pears and cranberries.
6. Once is fully blended, move to the prepared baking dish.
7. Spread the topping evenly over the fruit.
8. Bake for about half an hour.
9. Disperse chocolate chips out at the top.
10. Cook for another 10 minutes.
11. Have with ice cream.

Nutrition:

Calories: 128 Cal

Fat: 6.6 g

Carbs: 15 g

Fiber: 0.7 g

Protein: 2 g

Crunchy Chocolate Chip Coconut Macadamia Nut Cookies

Preparation Time: 10 Minutes

Cooking Time: 10 Minutes

Servings: 10

Ingredients:

- 1 cup yogurt
- 1 cup yogurt
- 1/2 tsp. baking soda
- 1/2 tsp. salt
- 1 tbsp. of butter, softened
- 1 cup firmly packed brown sugar
- 1/2 cup sugar
- 1 large egg
- 1/2 cup semi-sweet chocolate chips
- 1/2 cup sweetened flaked coconut
- 1/2 cup coarsely chopped dry-roasted macadamia nuts
- 1/2 cup raisins

Directions:

1. Preheat the oven to 325ºf.
2. In a little bowl, whisk together the flour, oats and baking soda and salt, then place aside.
3. In your mixer bowl, mix the butter/sugar/egg mix.
4. Mix in the flour/oats mix until just combined and stir into the chocolate chips, raisins, nuts and coconut.
5. Place outsized bits on a parchment-lined cookie sheet.
6. Bake for 1-3 minutes before biscuits are only barely golden brown.
7. Remove from the oven and then leave the cookie sheets to cool at least 10 minutes.

Nutrition:

Calories: 243 Cal

Fat: 12.6 g

Carbs: 30.3 g

Fiber: 1.5 g

Protein: 4.4 g

Ultimate Chocolate Chip Cookie N' Oreo Fudge Brownie Bar

Preparation Time: 15 Minutes

Cooking Time: 60 Minutes

Servings: 10

Ingredients:

- 1 cup (2 sticks) butter, softened
- 1 cup granulated sugar
- 3/4 cup light brown sugar
- 2 large eggs
- 1 tablespoon pure vanilla extract
- 2 ½ cups all-purpose flour
- 1 tsp. baking soda
- 1 tsp. lemon
- 2 cups (12 oz.) milk chocolate chips
- 1 package double-stuffed Oreo
- 1 family-size (9×1 3) brownie mixture
- 1/4 cup hot fudge topping

Directions:

1. Preheat oven to 350 degrees F.
2. First, cream the butter and sugars in a bowl using an electric mixer at medium speed for 35 minutes.
3. Add the vanilla and eggs and mix well to combine thoroughly. In a separate bowl, whisk together the salt, flour and baking soda then slowly incorporate it in the mixer until everything is combined.
4. Stir in chocolate chips.
5. Spread the cookie dough at the bottom of a 9×1-3 baking dish that is wrapped with wax paper and then coated with cooking spray.
6. Shirt with a coating of Oreos. Mix brownie mix, adding an optional 1/4 cup of hot fudge directly into the mixture.
7. Stir the brownie batter within the cookie-dough and Oreos.
8. Cover with a foil and bake it at 350 degrees F for 30 minutes.
9. Remove foil and continue baking for another 15 25 minutes.
10. Let cool before cutting on brownies. They may be gooey while warm but will also set up perfectly once chilled.

Nutrition:

Calories: 490 Cal

Fat: 21.9 g

Carbs: 69 g

Fiber: 1.5 g

Protein: 5.5 g

Radish green pesto

Preparation Time: 15 Minutes

Cooking Time: 60 Minutes

Servings: 10

Ingredients:

- 2 handfuls
- fresh radish leaf (from 1–2 bunch of radishes in organic quality)
- 1 garlic
- 30 g pine nuts (2 tbsp)
- 30 g parmesan (1 piece; 30% fat in dry matter)
- 100 ml olive oil
- salt
- pepper
- 1 tsp lemon juice

Directions:

1. Wash the radish leaves and shake them dry. Peel and chop the garlic.
2. Roast pine nuts in a hot pan without fat over medium heat for 3 minutes. Grate the Parmesan finely.
3. Puree the radish leaves, garlic, pine nuts and the oil with a hand blender. Mix in the Parmesan. Season with salt, pepper and lemon juice.

Watercress smoothie

Preparation Time: 15 Minutes

Cooking Time: 60 Minutes

Servings: 10

Ingredients:

- 150 g watercress
- 1 small onion
- ½ cucumber
- 1 tbsp lemon juice
- 200 ml mineral water
- salt
- pepper
- 4 tbsp crushed ice

Directions:

1. Wash and spin dry watercress; put some sheets aside for the garnish.
2. Peel the onion and cut it into small cubes. Wash the cucumber half, halve lengthways and cut the pulp into tiny cubes; Set aside 4 tablespoons of cucumber cubes.
3. Puree the remaining cucumber cubes with cress, onion cubes, lemon juice, mineral water and ice in a blender.
4. Season the smoothie with salt and pepper, pour into 2 glasses and sprinkle with cucumber cubes and cress leaves.

Melon and spinach juice with cinnamon

Preparation Time: 15 Minutes

Cooking Time: 60 Minutes

Servings: 10

Ingredients:

- 350 g small honeydew melon (0.5 small honeydew melons)
- 250 g young tender spinach leaves
- 1 PC cinnamon stick (approx. 1 cm)
- nutmeg

Directions:

1. Core the melon with a teaspoon. First cut the melon into wedges, then cut the pulp from the skin and roughly dice.

2. Clean the spinach and wash thoroughly in a bowl of water. Renew the water several times until it remains clear.
3. Using a small sharp knife, scrape thin strips off the cinnamon stick.
4. Squeeze the spinach lightly; Put back a leaflet and a small stem for the garnish as you like. Juice the rest with the melon in a juicer and pour it into a glass with ice cubes. Rub a little nutmeg over it, garnish with cinnamon and possibly with the spinach set aside and enjoy immediately.

Christmas cocktail - vegan eggnog

Ingredients:

- 1 cup cashew nuts
- 1 cup soy or almond milk
- 2-3 glasses of water
- about 5 pieces of dates (more if you like sweeter drinks)
- 2-3 scoops of brandy or whiskey
- 1 tablespoon lemon juice (optional, to taste)
- 1-2 teaspoons cinnamon
- ½ teaspoons ground anise
- ½ teaspoons ground ginger
- 2 pinches nutmeg
- pinch of salt
- Process

Directions:

1. Pour dates and cashews with boiling water and leave to soak for 20 minutes. Transfer the remaining ingredients to the blender dish and finally add the drained nuts and dates.
2. Mix thoroughly in a high-speed blender for a few minutes, until a thick and creamy cocktail without lumps is formed. If your blender can't do it, mix

the cashews with water first and strain them with gauze.
3. Season the cocktail with more lemon juice and salt to tasteand if you prefer sweeter drinks, add 2-3 pieces of dates. Serve it chilled with a pinch of cinnamon.

Orange and mandarin liqueur

Preparation Time: 15 Minutes

Cooking Time: 60 Minutes

Servings: 10

Ingredients:

- 2 large oranges
- 2 tangerines
- 1 small lemon
- 300 g white sugar candy
- 1 stick of vanilla
- 50 ml of orange juice
- 250 ml double grain

Directions:

1. Put the sugar candy in a bottle or a screw-top jar.
2. Pour the citrus into small pieces and remove the skin.
3. Pour in the orange juice.
4. Add the vanilla stick.
5. Baste with the double grain
6. Fill up to the top of the bottle if desired.
7. Close the bottle.
8. Shake daily until the sugar candy has dissolved.
9. After 2 - 3 weeks pour the liqueur through a sieve.
10. Pour it back into the bottle.

Cucumber-apple-banana shake

Preparation Time: 15 Minutes

Cooking Time: 60 Minutes

Servings: 10

Ingredients:

- 1 lemon
- 1 banana
- 4th sour apples (e.g. granny smith)
- 1 bunch parsley
- ½ cucumber
- mineral water to fill up
- 10 dice ice cubes

Directions:

1. Halve the lemon and squeeze out the juice. Peel and dice the banana. Clean, wash, quarter the apples, remove the core, dice the pulp. Mix the apples with the banana cubes and lemon juice.
2. Wash parsley, shake dry and chop. Clean, peel and halve the cucumber, coreand cut into bite-size pieces. Put 3 pieces of cucumber on 4 wooden skewers.
3. Puree the remaining pieces of cucumber with fruit, parsley and ice in a blender. Spread over 4 glasses, fill up with mineral water to the desired consistency and garnish with 1 cucumber skewer each.

Kefir avocado shake with herbs

Preparation Time: 15 Minutes

Cooking Time: 60 Minutes

Servings: 10

Ingredients:

- 2 stems dill
- 2 stems parsley
- straws of chives
- 1 avocado
- 1 tsp honey
- 1 splash lime juice
- 4 ice cubes
- 300 ml kefir chilled
- salt
- 1 pinch wasabi powder

Directions:

1. Spray the herbs, pat dry, pluck and cut roughly except for a few dill tips for the garnish.
2. Peel, halve, core and cut the avocado into pieces. Puree with the herbs, honey, lime juice, ice cubes and kefir in a blender until creamy.
3. Season the smoothie with salt and wasabi and pour into glasses. Serve garnished with dill tips.

Mandarin liqueur

Preparation Time: 15 Minutes

Cooking Time: 60 Minutes

Servings: 10

Ingredients:

- 2 large oranges
- 2 tangerines
- 1 small lemon
- 300 g white sugar candy
- 1 stick of vanilla
- 50 ml of orange juice
- 250 ml double grain

Directions:

1. Put the sugar candy in a bottle or a screw-top jar.
2. Pour the citrus into small pieces and remove the skin.
3. Pour in the orange juice.
4. Add the vanilla stick.

5. Baste with the double grain and fill up to the top of the bottle if desired.
6. Close the bottle.
7. Shake daily until the sugar candy has dissolved.
8. After 2 - 3 weeks pour the liqueur through a sieve and pour it back into the bottle.

Pear and lime marmalade

Ingredients: for 1.5 l jam

- 3-4 untreated limes
- 1 kg ripe pears
- 500 g jam sugar 2: 1

Preparation

1. Wash 2 limes and grate dry.
2. Peel the peels thinly with the zest ripper.
3. Then cut all limes in half and squeeze them out. Measure out 100 ml of lime juice.
4. Wash and peel the pears, remove the core and then quarter them. Weigh 900 g of pulp.
5. Then puree the pears together with the lime juice.
6. Now put the pear puree together with the lime peels and the jellied sugar in a saucepan.
7. Bring all ingredients to the boil together.
8. Simmer for 4 minutes, stirring, taking care not to burn anything.
9. Make a gelation test with a small blob on a cold saucer. If this becomes solid in a short time, the jam is ready Remove any foam that may have formed with a spade, but you can also simply stir it in.
10. Then pour the hot mass into hot rinsed jars, close and let stand upside down.

Healthy green shot

Preparation Time: 15 Minutes

Cooking Time: 60 Minutes

Servings: 10

Ingredients:

- 2 pears
- 3 green apples (e.g. granny smith)
- 3 sticks celery
- 60 g organic ginger
- 1 bunch parsley (20 g)
- 3 kiwi fruit
- 2 limes
- 1 tsp turmeric

Directions:

1. Wash pears, apples, celery, ginger and parsley and cut into pieces. Halve the kiwi fruit and remove the pulp with a spoon. Halve limes and squeeze out juice.
2. Put the pears, apples, kiwi, celery, ginger and parsley in the juicer and squeeze out the juice.
3. Mix freshly squeezed juice with the lime juice and season with turmeric. Serve the mixture as shots immediately or freeze it in portions.

Spinach kiwi smoothie bowl

Preparation Time: 15 Minutes

Cooking Time: 60 Minutes

Servings: 10

Ingredients:

- 1 green apple
- 2 kiwi fruit
- 300 g bananas (2 bananas)
- 100 g baby spinach

- 1 lemon
- 6 g chia seeds (2 tsp)
- 20 g grated coconut (2 tbsp)

Directions:

1. Clean, wash, core and chop the apple. Peel and cut the kiwis and bananas and put half aside. Wash the spinach and put some leaves aside. Halve the lemon and squeeze out the juice.
2. Put half of the fruit, spinach and lemon juice in a blender and mash finely. Divide the smoothie into 4 bowls.
3. Put the remaining pieces of fruit as a topping on the smoothie bowls. Sprinkle with chia seeds and grated coconut and serve with the remaining spinach leaves.

Avocado smoothie with basil

Preparation Time: 15 Minutes

Cooking Time: 60 Minutes

Servings: 10

Ingredients:

- 2 kiwi fruit
- 1 yellow-peeled apple
- 200 g honeydew melon meat
- 1 avocado
- 1 green chili pepper
- 20 g basil (1 handful)
- 20 g arugula (0.25 bunch)
- 1 tbsp sprouts (suitable for raw consumption)

Directions:

1. Peel and slice the kiwi fruit. Wash, quarter and core the apple and cut the quarters into slices. Cut the melon meat into pieces. Peel, core and cut avocado into pieces. Wash the chili pepper and cut it into rings. Wash the basil and rocket and shake dry. Shower sprouts in a sieve.
2. Put all prepared ingredients in a blender and mash them finely. Add about 100 ml of cold water and serve in 4 glasses.

Gooseberry buttermilk drink

Preparation Time: 15 Minutes

Cooking Time: 60 Minutes

Servings: 10

Ingredients:

- 300 g gooseberries
- 2 bananas
- 600 ml buttermilk
- 30 g honey (2 tbsp)
- 4 small stems of mint
- ice cubes

Directions:

1. Wash and clean gooseberries and drain well. Set some berries aside for the garnish.
2. Peel and slice bananas. Puree together with gooseberries and 200 ml buttermilk. Add the remaining buttermilk and honey and mix until frothy.
3. Fill 4 glasses about halfway with ice cubes and spread the drink on them.
4. Wash the mint, shake it dry and spread it with the rest of the gooseberries on the drinks.

Blackberry and vanilla smoothie

Preparation Time: 15 Minutes

Cooking Time: 60 Minutes

Servings: 10

Ingredients:

- 500 g blackberry
- 1 vanilla bean
- 1 tsp lemon juice
- 700 ml buttermilk (ice cold)
- 80 g lean quark (4 tbsp)
- 40 g cashews
- 80 ml whipped cream

Directions:

1. Wash and drain blackberries.
2. Cut the vanilla pod lengthways, scrape out the pulp and puree creamy with blackberries, lemon juice, buttermilk, curd cheese and cashew nuts in a blender.
3. Whip the cream. Pour smoothie into 4 glasses and garnish with cream

Dijon Celery Salad

Preparation Time: 10 minutes

Cooking Time: 0 minutes

Servings: 4

Ingredients:

- 5 teaspoons stevia
- ½ cup lemon juice
- 1/3 cup dijon mustard
- 2/3 cup olive oil
- black pepper to the taste
- 2 apples, cored, peeled and cubed
- 1 bunch celery and leaves, roughly chopped
- ¾ cup walnuts, chopped

Directions:

1. In a salad bowl, mix celery and its leaves with apple pieces and walnuts.

2. Add black pepper, lemon juice, mustard, stevia and olive oil.
3. Whisk well, add to your salad, toss.
4. Divide into small cups and serve as a snack.

Nutrition:

Calories: 125 Cal

Fat: 2 g

Carbohydrates: 7 g

Protein: 7 g

Fiber: 2 g

Dill Bell Pepper Snack Bowls

Preparation Time: 10 minutes

Cooking Time: 0 minutes

Servings: 4

Ingredients:

- 2 tablespoons dill, chopped
- 1 yellow onion, chopped
- 1-pound multicolored bell peppers, cut into halves, seeded and cut into thin strips
- 3 tablespoons olive oil
- 2 and ½ tablespoons white vinegar
- Black pepper to the taste

Directions:

1. In a salad bowl, mix bell peppers with onion, dill, pepper, oil and vinegar, toss to coat, divide into small bowls and serve as a snack.

Nutrition:

Calories: 120 Cal

Fat: 3 g

Carbohydrates: 2 g

Protein: 3 g

Fiber: 3 g

Cinnamon Apple Chips

Preparation Time: 10 minutes

Cooking Time: 2 hours

Servings: 4

Ingredients:

- Cooking spray
- 2 teaspoons cinnamon powder
- 2 apples, cored and thinly sliced

Directions:

1. Arrange apple slices on a lined baking sheet, spray them with cooking oil, sprinkle cinnamon, introduce in the oven and bake at 300 degrees F for 2 hours.
2. Divide into bowls and serve as a snack.

Nutrition:

Calories: 80 Cal

Fat: 0 g

Carbohydrates: 7 g

Protein: 4 g

Fiber: 3 g

Potato Bites

Preparation Time: 10 minutes

Cooking Time: 20 minutes

Servings: 3

Ingredients:

- 1 potato, sliced
- 2 bacon slices, already cooked and crumbled

- 1 small avocado, pitted and cubed
- Cooking spray

Directions:

1. Spread potato slices on a lined baking sheet, spray with cooking oil, introduce in the oven at 350 degrees F, bake for 20 minutes, arrange on a platter, top each slice with avocado and crumbled bacon and serve as a snack.

Nutrition:

Calories: 180 Cal

Fat: 4 g

Carbohydrates: 8 g

Protein: 6 g

Fiber: 1 g

Beans Snack Salad

Preparation Time: 10 minutes

Cooking Time: 0 minutes

Servings: 6

Ingredients:

- 2 cups tomatoes, chopped
- 2 cups cucumber, chopped
- 3 cups mixed greens
- 2 cups mung beans, sprouted
- 2 cups clover sprouts
- for the salad dressing:
- 1 tablespoon cumin, ground
- 1 cup dill, chopped
- 4 tablespoons lemon juice
- 1 avocado, pitted, peeled and roughly chopped
- 1 cucumber, roughly chopped

Directions:

2. In a salad bowl.

3. Mix tomatoes with 2 cups cucumber, greens, clover and mung sprouts.
4. In your blender, mix cumin with dill, lemon juice, 1 cucumber and avocado.
5. Blend well, add this to your salad, toss well and serve as a snack.

Nutrition:

Calories: 120 Cal

Fat: 0 g

Carbohydrates: 1 g

Protein: 6 g

Fiber: 2 g

Sprouts and Apple Snack Salad

Preparation Time: 10 minutes

Cooking Time: 0 minute

Servings: 4

Ingredients:

- 1-pound brussels sprouts, shredded
- 1 cup walnuts, chopped
- 1 apple, cored and cubed
- 1 red onion, chopped
- For the salad dressing:
- 3 tablespoons red vinegar
- 1 tablespoon mustard
- 1/2 cup olive oil
- 1 garlic clove, minced
- Black pepper to the taste

Directions:

1. In a salad bowl, mix sprouts with apple, onion and walnuts.
2. In another bowl, mix vinegar with mustard, oil, garlic and pepper, whisk well, add this to your salad, toss well and serve as a snack.

Nutrition:

Calories: 120 Cal

Fat: 2 g

Carbohydrates: 8 g

Protein: 6 g

Fiber: 2 g

Moroccan Leeks Snack Salad

Preparation Time: 10 minutes

Cooking Time: 0 minutes

Servings: 4

Ingredients:

- 1 bunch radishes, sliced
- 3 cups leeks, chopped
- 1 and ½ cups olives, pitted and sliced
- A pinch of turmeric powder
- Black pepper to the taste
- 2 tablespoons olive oil
- 1 cup cilantro, chopped

Directions:

1. In a bowl, mix radishes with leeks, olives and cilantro.
2. Add black pepper, oil and turmeric, toss to coat and serve as a snack.

Nutrition:

Calories: 120 Cal

Fat: 1 g

Carbohydrates: 8 g

Protein: 6 g

Fiber: 1 g

Celery and Raisins Snack Salad

Preparation Time: 10 minutes

Cooking Time: 0 minutes

Servings: 4

Ingredients:

- ½ cup raisins
- 4 cups celery, sliced
- ¼ cup parsley, chopped
- ½ cup walnuts, chopped
- Juice of ½ lemon
- 2 tablespoons olive oil
- Salt and black pepper to the taste

Directions:

1. In a salad bowl.
2. Mix celery with raisins, walnuts, parsley, lemon juice, oil and black pepper, toss
3. Divide into small cups and serve as a snack.

Nutrition:

Calories: 120 Cal

Fat: 1 g

Carbohydrates: 6 g

Protein: 5 g

Fiber: 2 g

Dijon Celery Salad

Preparation Time: 10 minutes

Cooking Time: 0 minutes

Servings: 4

Ingredients:

- 5 teaspoons stevia
- ½ cup lemon juice
- 1/3 cup Dijon mustard
- 2/3 cup olive oil
- Black pepper to the taste
- 2 apples, cored, peeled and cubed

- 1 bunch celery and leaves, roughly chopped
- ¾ cup walnuts, chopped

Directions:

1. In a salad bowl, mix celery and its leaves with apple pieces and walnuts.
2. Add black pepper, lemon juice, mustard, stevia and olive oil, whisk well, add to your salad, toss, divide into small cups and serve as a snack.

Nutrition:

Calories: 125 Cal

Fat: 2 g

Carbohydrates: 7 g

Protein: 7 g

Fiber: 2 g

Mozzarella Bars

Preparation Time: 10 minutes

Cooking Time: 40 minutes

Servings: 12

Ingredients:

- 1 big cauliflower head, riced
- ½ cup low-fat mozzarella cheese, shredded
- ¼ cup egg whites
- 1 teaspoon Italian seasoning
- Black pepper to the taste

Directions:

1. Spread the cauliflower rice on a lined baking sheet, cook in the oven at 375 degrees F for 20 minutes.
2. Transfer to a bowl, add black pepper, cheese, seasoning and egg whites.

3. Stir well, spread into a rectangle pan and press on the bottom.
4. Introduce in the oven at 375 degrees F, bake for 20 minutes, cut into 12 bars.
5. and serve as a snack.

Nutrition:

Calories: 140 Cal

Fat: 1 g

Carbohydrates: 6 g

Protein: 6 g

Fiber: 3 g

Baby Spinach Snack

Preparation Time: 10 minutes

Cooking Time: 10 min

Servings: 3

Ingredients:

- 2 cups baby spinach, washed
- A pinch of black pepper
- ½ tablespoon olive oil
- ½ teaspoon garlic powder

Directions:

1. Spread the baby spinach on a lined baking sheet, add oil, black pepper and garlic powder, toss a bit, introduce in the oven, bake at 350 degrees F for 10 minutes, divide into bowls and serve as a snack.

Nutrition:

Calories: 125 Cal

Fat: 4 g

Carbohydrates: 4 g

Protein: 2 g

Fiber: 1 g

Italian Veggie Salsa

Preparation Time: 10 minutes

Cooking Time: 10 minutes

Servings: 4

Ingredients:

- 2 red bell peppers, cut into medium wedges
- 3 zucchinis, sliced
- ½ cup garlic, minced
- 2 tablespoons olive oil
- A pinch of black pepper
- 1 teaspoon Italian seasoning

Directions:

1. Heat a pan with the oil over medium-high heat, add bell peppers and zucchini, toss and cook for 5 minutes.
2. Add garlic, black pepper and Italian seasoning, toss, cook for 5 minutes more, divide into small cups and serve as a snack.

Nutrition:

Calories: 132 g

Fat: 3 g

Carbohydrates: 7 g

Protein: 4 g

Fiber: 3 g

Black Bean Salsa

Preparation Time: 10 minutes

Cooking Time: 0 minutes

Servings: 6

Ingredients:

- 1 tablespoon coconut amino
- ½ teaspoon cumin, ground

- 1 cup canned black beans, no-salt-added, drained and rinsed
- 1 cup salsa
- 6 cups romaine lettuce leaves, torn
- ½ cup avocado, peeled, pitted and cubed

Directions:

1. In a bowl, combine the beans with the amino, cumin, salsa, lettuce and avocado, toss, divide into small bowls and serve as a snack

Nutrition:

Calories: 181 Cal

Fat: 4 g

Carbohydrates: 14 g

Protein: 7 g

Fiber: 7 g

Pumpkin Seeds Bowls

Preparation Time: 10 minutes

Cooking Time: 20 minutes

Servings: 6

Ingredients:

- ½ tablespoon chili powder
- ½ teaspoon cayenne pepper
- 2 cups pumpkin seeds
- 2 teaspoons lime juice

Directions:

1. Spread pumpkin seeds on a lined baking sheet.
2. Add lime juice, cayenne and chili powder, toss well, introduce in the oven.
3. Roast at 275 degrees F for 20 minutes.

4. Divide into small bowls and serve as a snack.

Nutrition:

Calories: 170 Cal

Fat: 2 g

Carbohydrates: 12 g

Protein: 6 g

Fiber: 7 g

Eggplant Salsa

Preparation Time: 10 minutes

Cooking Time: 10 minutes

Servings: 4

Ingredients:

- 1 And ½ Cups Tomatoes, Chopped
- 3 Cups Eggplant, Cubed
- A Drizzle Of Olive Oil
- 2 Teaspoons Capers
- 6 Ounces Green Olives, Pitted And Sliced
- 4 Garlic Cloves, Minced
- 2 Teaspoons Balsamic Vinegar
- 1 Tablespoon Basil, Chopped
- Black Pepper To The Taste

Directions:

1. Heat A Pan With The Oil Over Medium-High Heat, Add Eggplant, Stirand Cook For 5 Minutes. Add Tomatoes, Capers, Olives, Garlic, Vinegar, Basil And Black Pepper, Toss, Cook For 5 Minutes More, Divide Into Small Cupsand Serve Cold.

Nutrition:

Calories: 120 Cal

Fat: 6 g

Carbohydrates: 9 g

Protein: 7 g

Fiber: 5 g

Date Nut Bread

Preparation Time: 30 minutes

Cooking Time: 4-6 hours

Servings: 4-6

Ingredients:

- ¾ cup Medjool dates
- 1 ¼ cup All-Purpose flour
- 2 teaspoon baking powder
- ¼ teaspoon baking soda
- ½ teaspoon salt
- ½ cup sugar
- ¾ cup milk
- 1 egg, slightly beaten
- 1 tablespoon orange peel, grated
- 1 tablespoon coconut oil, melted
- ¼ cup buckwheat flour
- 1 cup walnuts, chopped

Directions:

2. Place the dates on a chopping block and sprinkle 1 tablespoon of All-Purpose flour over them. Dip a knife into the flour and chop the dates finely. Flour the knife often to keep the cut-up fruit from sticking together.
3. Sift the remaining All-Purpose flour, baking powder, baking soda, salt and sugar into a large bowl.
4. In a separate bowl, combine the milk, egg, orange peel and oil.
5. Add the buckwheat flour to the flour mixture, mix well and gently fold in the dates, along with any flour left on the cutting block and the walnuts.
6. Pour in the liquid ingredients and mix until just combined.
7. Transfer dough into a well-greased and floured baking unit. Cover and place in the slow cooker
8. Use a toothpick or small amount of twisted aluminum foil to prop the crockpot lid open a tiny fraction to allow steam to escape.
9. Cook on high for 4 to 6 hours. Cool on a rack for 10 minutes. Serve warm or cold.
10. Do NOT lift the crockpot lid while the bread is baking.

Nutrition:

Calories: 70 Cal

Fat:1 g

Carbohydrates: 15 g

Protein: 1 g

Fiber: 1 g

Strawberry Rhubarb Crisp

Preparation Time: 10 minutes

Cooking Time: 45 minutes

Servings: 6-8

Ingredients:

- 1 cup white sugar
- ½ cup buckwheat flour + 3 tablespoons
- 3 cups strawberries, sliced
- 3 cups rhubarb, diced
- ½ lemon, juiced
- 1 cup packed brown sugar
- 1 cup coconut oil, melted
- ¾ cup rolled oats
- ¼ cup buckwheat groats
- ¼ cup walnuts, chopped

Directions:

1. Preheat oven to 375 degrees F
2. In a large bowl, mix white sugar, 3 tablespoons flour, strawberries, rhubarb and lemon juice. Place the mixture in a 9x13 inch baking dish.
3. In a separate bowl, mix ½ cup flour, brown sugar, coconut oil, oats, buckwheat groats and walnuts until crumbly. You may want to use a pastry blender for this. Crumble on top of the rhubarb and strawberry mixture.
4. Bake 45 minutes in the preheated oven, or until crisp and lightly browned.

Nutrition:

Calories: 240 Cal

Fat: 7 g

Carbohydrates: 42 g

Protein: 2 g

Fiber: 3 g

Avocado Smoothie

Preparation Time: 5 Minutes

Cooking Time: 5 Minutes

Servings: 2

Ingredients:

- 1 cup Coconut Milk, preferably full-fat
- 1 cup Ice
- 3 cups Baby Spinach
- 1 Banana, frozen & quartered
- 1/2 cup pineapple chunks, frozen
- 1/2 of 1 Avocado, smooth

Directions:

1. First, place ice, pineapple chunks, pineapple chunks, banana, avocado, baby spinach in the blender pitcher.
2. Now, press the 'extract' button.

3. Finally, transfer to a serving glass.
4. To make it more nutritious and filling, you can even add banana to it.

Nutrition:

130 calories

Tofu Smoothie

Preparation Time: 5 Minutes

Cooking Time: 5 Minutes

Servings: 2

Ingredients:

- 1 Banana, sliced & frozen
- 3/4 cup Almond Milk
- 2 tbsp. Peanut Butter
- 1/2 cup Yoghurt, plain & low-fat
- 1/2 cup Tofu, soft & silken
- 1/3 cup Dates, chopped

Directions:

1. First, place tofu, banana, dates, yogurt, peanut butter and almond milk in the blender pitcher.
2. After that, press the 'smoothie' button.
3. Finally, transfer to serving glass and enjoy it.
4. Tip: You can try adding herbs to your preference.

Nutrition:

Calories: 119 Sugar: 13

Sodium: 31 Fat: 2 Carbohydrates: 22

Fiber: 3 Protein: 5

Carrot Strawberry Smoothie

Preparation Time: 5 Minutes

Cooking Time: 5 Minutes

Servings: 2

Ingredients:

- 1/3 cup Bell Pepper, diced
- 1 cup Carrot Juice, chilled
- 1 cup Mango, diced
- 1 cup Strawberries, unsweetened & frozen

Directions:

1. To start with, place strawberries, bell pepper and mango in the blender pitcher.
2. After that, pulse it a few times.
3. Pour the carrot juice into it.
4. Finally, press the 'smoothie' button.
5. Tip: You can try adding pineapple chunks to it for enhanced flavour.

Nutrition:

70 calories

Green Smoothie

Preparation Time: 5 Minutes

Cooking Time: 5 Minutes

Servings: 3 to 4

Ingredients:

- 1/4 cup Baby Spinach
- 1/2 cup Ice
- 1/4 cup Kale
- 1/2 cup Pineapple Chunks
- 1/2 cup Coconut Water
- 1/2 cup mango, diced
- 1/2 Banana, diced

Directions:

1. Begin by placing all the ingredients needed to make the smoothie in the blender pitcher.

2. Now, press the 'extract' button.
3. Transfer the smoothie into the serving glass.

Nutrition:

Calories: 207 Carbohydrates: 33 grams Fat: 2 grams

Protein: 15 grams Sodium: 73 milligrams Sugar: 25 grams

Fiber: 5 grams Cholesterol: 4 milligrams

Yoghurt & Fruit Jam Parfait

Preparation Time: 5 Minutes

Cooking Time: 5 Minutes

Servings: 6

Ingredients:

- 3 cups Mixed Berries
- 1 tbsp. Lemon Juice
- 7/8 cup Honey
- 2 tsp. Fruit Pectin
- 1 cup Granola
- 3 cups Greek Yoghurt

Directions:

1. For making this healthy jam, you need to place the mixed berries, honey, lemon juice and pectin in the blender pitcher.
2. Pulse the mixture 3 to 4 times and then press the 'sauce/ dip' button.
3. Now, transfer the jam to a safe heat container and then place it in the refrigerator for 2 to 3 hours.
4. Once the jam is chilled, layer 1/3 cup of the Greek Yoghurt into the bottom of the parfait glass.
5. After that, spoon in a jam into it and then add the granola.
6. Serve immediately.

Tip: If you don't want to use honey, you can use 1 cup of granulated sugar.

Nutrition: 154 calories

Kiwi Smoothie

Preparation Time: 5 Minutes

Cooking Time: 5 Minutes

Servings: 3

Ingredients:

- 1/4 of 1 Avocado, ripe & pitted
- 1/4 cup Ice
- 1/4 cup Coconut Water
- 3/4 cup Kale Leaves
- 1/2 cm Ginger, fresh & peeled
- 2 Kiwis, quartered
- 1 Date pitted & halved
- 1 tsp. Lime Juice

Directions:

1. First, place ice, kale leaves, avocado, dates, kiwis, lime juice, ginger and coconut water in the blender pitcher.
2. Then, press the 'smoothie' button.
3. Finally, transfer to a serving glass and enjoy it.

Nutrition:

Calories: 268.0 Total Fat: 2.3 g Cholesterol: 40.0 mg

Sodium: 141.2 mg Total Carbs: 34.3 g Dietary Fiber: 6.0 g Protein: 27.9 g

Pineapple Kale Smoothie

Preparation Time: 5 Minutes

Cooking Time: 5 Minutes

Servings: 3

Ingredients:

- 3/4 cup Kale leaves
- 1 cup Pineapple, fresh & chopped into chunks
- 1/4 cup Ice
- 3/4 cup Coconut Water
- 1/4 of 1 Avocado, ripe & pitted
- 1/2 of 1 Lime
- 1 Date pitted & halved

Directions:

1. For making this bright, tasty smoothie, place ice, kale leaves, avocado, date, coconut water, lime and pineapple in the blender pitcher.
2. After that, press the 'smoothie' button.
3. Finally, transfer the smoothie to a serving glass and enjoy it.
4. For a richer smoothie, you can try substituting coconut water with light coconut milk.

Nutrition:

Calories: 266.3 Total Fat: 0.6 g Cholesterol: 0.0 mg

Sodium: 34.9 mg Total Carbs: 68.6 g Dietary Fiber: 8.8 g Protein: 4.0 g

Antioxidant Smoothie

Preparation Time: 5 Minutes

Cooking Time: 5 Minutes

Servings: 3

Ingredients:

- 1/2 cup Celery Stalk, halved
- 1/3 cup Watermelon, chopped into chunks
- 1/4 cup Ice
- 1/8 cup Red Cabbage, chopped
- 1/2 cup Blueberries

- 1/2 cup Pomegranate Juice
- 1/2 of 1 Apple, unpeeled & halved

Directions:

1. Begin by placing ice, red cabbage, celery stalk, apple, blueberries and watermelon in the blender pitcher.
2. Now, select the 'smoothie' button.
3. Finally, transfer the smoothie to the serving glass and enjoy it.

Nutrition:

Calories: 225.3 Total Fat: 9.1 g

Cholesterol: 10.0 mg Sodium: 135.5 mg

Total Carbs: 29.7 g

Dietary Fiber: 7.2 g

Protein: 9.1 g

Carrot Beetroot Smoothie

Preparation Time: 5 Minutes

Cooking Time: 5 Minutes

Servings: 3

Ingredients:

- 1/2 of 1 Beet, small & halved
- 3/4 cup Water
- 1/2 cup Ice
- 1 Celery Stalk
- 1/2 of 1 Lemon
- 1/2 of 1 Carrot, halved
- 1/2 cm Ginger, fresh & peeled
- 1/2 of 1 Orange, halved

Directions:

1. To start with, place ice, carrot, beet, celery stalk, lemon, ginger, orange and water in the blender pitcher.
2. Then select the 'smoothie' button.

3. Finally, transfer the smoothie to the serving glass.
4. Tip: For a more vibrant smoothie, you can try substituting coconut water with light coconut milk.

Nutrition:

Calories: 169.7 Total Fat: 1.0 g Cholesterol: 0.0 mg

Sodium: 112.3 mg Total Carbs: 38.3 g Dietary Fiber: 3.6 g Protein: 3.7 g

Black Tea Cake

Preparation Time: 10 minutes.

Cooking Time: 35 minutes.

Servings: 8

Ingredients:

- 6 tablespoons black tea powder
- 2 cups almond milk, warmed up
- 1 cup avocado oil
- 2 cups stevia
- 4 eggs
- 2 teaspoons vanilla extract
- 3 and ½ cups almond flour
- 1 teaspoon baking soda
- 3 teaspoons baking powder

Directions:

1. In a bowl, combine the almond milk with the oil, stevia and the rest of the ingredients and whisk well.
2. Pour this into a cake pan lined with parchment paper, introduce in the oven at 350ºF and bake for 35 minutes.
3. Leave the cake to cool down, slice and serve.

Nutrition:

Carbs: 6.5g.

Protein: 5.4g.

Green Tea and Vanilla Cream

Preparation Time: 2 hours.

Cooking Time: 0 minutes.

Servings: 4

Ingredients:

- 14 ounces almond milk, hot
- 2 tablespoons green tea powder
- 14 ounces heavy cream
- 3 tablespoons stevia
- 1 teaspoon vanilla extract
- 1 teaspoon gelatin powder

Directions:

1. In a bowl, combine the almond milk with the green tea powder and the rest of the ingredients, whisk well, cool down, divide into cups and keep in the fridge for 2 hours before serving.

Nutrition:

Calories: 120

Fat: 3g.

Carbs: 7g.

Protein: 4g.

120. Figs Pie

Preparation Time: 10 minutes.

Cooking Time: 1 hour.

Servings: 8

Ingredients:

- ½ cup stevia
- 6 figs, cut into quarters
- ½ teaspoon vanilla extract
- 1 cup almond flour
- 4 eggs, whisked

Directions:

1. Spread the figs on the bottom of a springform pan lined with parchment paper.
2. In a bowl, combine the other ingredients, whisk and pour over the figs.
3. Bake at 375ºF for 1 hour, flip the pie upside down when it's done and serve.

Nutrition:

Calories: 200

Fat: 4.4g.

Carbs: 7.6g.

Protein: 8g.

Cherry Cream

Preparation Time: 2 hours.

Cooking Time: 0 minutes.

Servings: 4

Ingredients:

- 2 cups cherries, pitted and chopped
- 1 cup almond milk
- ½ cup whipping cream
- 3 eggs, whisked
- 1/3 cup stevia
- 1 teaspoon lemon juice
- ½ teaspoon vanilla extract

Directions:

1. In your food processor, combine the cherries with the milk and the rest of the ingredients, pulse well, divide into cups and keep in the fridge for 2 hours before serving.

Nutrition:

Calories: 200

Fat: 4.5g.

Carbs: 5.6g.

Protein: 3.4g.

Strawberries Cream

Preparation Time: 10 minutes.

Cooking Time: 20 minutes.

Servings: 4

Ingredients:

- ½ cup stevia
- 2 pounds strawberries, chopped
- 1 cup almond milk
- Zest of 1 lemon, grated
- ½ cup heavy cream
- 3 egg yolks, whisked

Directions:

2. Heat up a pan with the milk over medium-high heat, add the stevia and the rest of the ingredients, whisk well, simmer for 20 minutes, divide into cups and serve cold.

Nutrition:

Calories: 152

Fat: 4.4g.

Carbs: 5.1g.

Protein: 0.8g.

A 21 Day Sirtfood Diet Meal Plan

DAYS	BREAKFAST	LUNCH	DINNER	DESSERT
1.	Kale Scramble	King Prawn Stir-fry & Soba	Lamb Chops with Kale	Italian Veggie Salsa
2.	Buckwheat Porridge	Miso Caramelized Tofu	Shrimp with Kale	Black Bean Salsa
3.	Salmon & Kale Omelet	Sirtfood Cauliflower Couscous & Turkey Steak	Chicken & Veggies with Buckwheat Noodles	Pumpkin Seeds Bowls
4.	Moroccan Spiced Eggs	Mushroom & Tofu Scramble	Beef & Kale Salad	Eggplant Salsa
5.	Chilaquiles with Gochujang	Prawn & Chili Pak Choi	Prawns with Asparagus	Date Nut Bread
6.	Twice Baked Breakfast Potatoes	Sirtfood Granola	Turkey Satay Skewer	Strawberry Rhubarb Crisp
7.	Sirt Muesli	Tomato Frittata	Salmon & Capers	Avocado Smoothie
8.	Mushroom Scramble Eggs	Horseradish Flaked Salmon Fillet & Kale	Chicken Casserole	Tofu Smoothie

9.	Smoked Salmon Omelets	Indulgent Yoghurt	Veal Cabbage Rolls – Smarter with Capers, Garlic and Caraway Seeds	Carrot Strawberry Smoothie
10.	Date and Walnut Porridge	Tuna Salad	Fragrant Asian Hotspot	Green Smoothie
11.	Beef Stroganoff French Bread Toast	Chicken & Bean Casserole	Tofu Thai Curry	Yoghurt & Fruit Jam Parfait
12.	Classic French Toast	Mussels in Red Wine Sauce	Beans & Kale Soup	Kiwi Smoothie
13.	Avocado and Kale Omelet	Tuna and Kale	Lentils & Greens Soup	Pineapple Kale Smoothie
14.	Easy Egg-White Muffins	Lemongrass Mix	Asian Slaw	Antioxidant Smoothie
15.	Avocado Eggs with Toast	Scallops with Almonds and Mushrooms	Egg Fried Buckwheat	Carrot Beetroot Smoothie
16.	Baked Oatmeal	Scallops and Sweet Potatoes	Aromatic Ginger Turmeric Buckwheat	Black Tea Cake
17.	Sirt cereal	Salmon and Shrimp Salad	Kale and Corn Succotash	Green Tea and Vanilla Cream
18.	Sirt breakfast bar	Shrimp, Tomato and Dates Salad	Asian King Prawn Stir-Fry with	Cherry Cream

			Buckwheat Noodles	
19.	Sirt cocoa pops	Salmon and Watercress Salad	Greek Salad Skewers	Strawberries Cream
20.	Sirt fruit bowl	Tuna and Tomatoes	Sirtfood Couscous	Mozzarella Bars
21.	Grilled sausages with fried Onions and scrambled eggs with herbs	Spinach and Kale Mix	Caramelized Tofu	Baby Spinach Snack

Conclusion

Thank you for making it to the end. Everything you have learned about the Sirtfood Diet, the important question, at least for many people, is whether or not it is worth your time and effort.

Though this trial's findings have proven to be quite promising, other experts have noted certain limitations of the study that could have been improved upon if subsequent follow-up trials had been conducted. Some of the most prominent limitations identified include the following:

- Lack of control group to as serve as baseline and reference point;
- Having 40 participants only, which is a relatively small sample size; and
- Potential bias among the participants since they have been identified as health-conscious individuals.

These limitations, while not conclusive, somehow weaken the foundations of the Sirtfood Diet. Some health experts even argue that much like other types of diets, Sirtfood Diet could help its followers lose weight by imposing caloric limits for a certain period.

While restrictive eating can be helpful and effective to a certain extent, several studies have highlighted the negative impacts that this practice causes. If you have already tried doing diets that are centered on regular fasting, then you would have experienced mood swings, sudden binges to compensate for the lack of food, loss of muscle mass and strength, and even depression.

Granted that you will not be required to undergo special exercise routines or to cut back on different types of food, you would still have to be mindful of what you eat and drink while you are on the Sirtfood diet. Nonetheless, this level of leniency that this diet offers to attract a lot of people who do not want to give up a lot of things for the sake of looking and feeling better.

So, what's the verdict on the Sirtfood Diet?

If you are willing to live through its drawbacks to reap its benefits and enjoy its advantages over other weight loss plans, then go ahead with your plans to follow this diet.

Furthermore, the majority of the top sirtfoods are fruits, vegetables, and plant-based foods. When combined with the right amount of proteins and carbohydrates in your daily meals, then you cannot go wrong by eating more of them than you usually do. Just remember to keep your red wine, caffeine, and dark chocolate in moderation, though, to avoid causing unintentional harm to your body.

Finally, as a rule of thumb, you should not put your 100% trust on a diet that has promises that sound a bit too good to be true. Set realistic expectations based on your current situation in life. Not everyone can live like Adele and the other celebrity endorsers of the Sirtfood Diet. Before you do this diet, think carefully. Chances are it might have a negative effect on your health if you don't follow the diet correctly. Think before you do anything. Sirtfood Diet is not that bad as long as you follow the plan correctly.

I hope you have learned something!